Addiction Inbox

Cutting-Edge Research on Drugs and Dependence

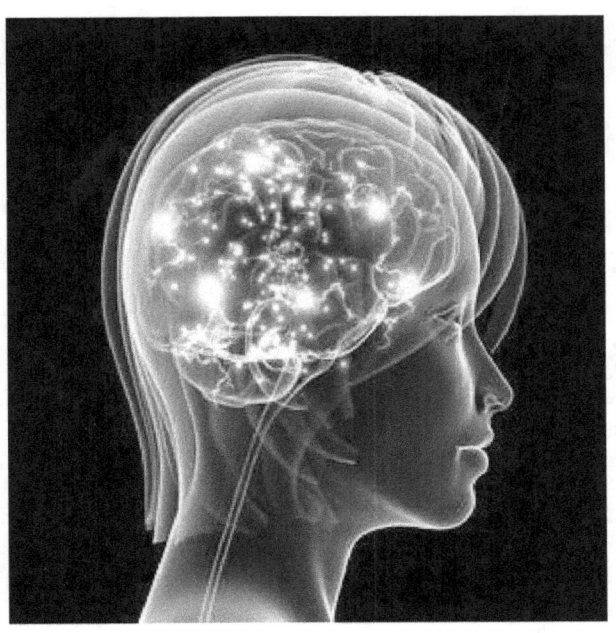

Dirk Hanson

For Drew, at last.

Books by Dirk Hanson

THE NEW ALCHEMISTS

THE SEVENTH LEVEL

THE CHEMICAL CAROUSEL

Introduction

What do we mean when we talk about addiction? This anthology of articles is designed to bring multiple perspectives to bear on that question, a pursuit made possible by the recent explosion of research on the scientific underpinnings of drug and alcohol addiction. In this collection of posts from my blog, Addiction Inbox, you'll meet some of the researchers, and some of the research. You'll learn about the new synthetic stimulant drugs now flooding American grey markets. And you'll hear about some of the best recent books on addiction and recovery.

My blog covers health studies about drugs, addiction and alcoholism, including the most recent scientific and medical findings—plus interviews, book reviews, and whatever else catches my interest. Readers familiar with Addiction Inbox may find some favorites, and hopefully some interesting ones they may have missed. For those unfamiliar with Addiction Inbox, this collection serves as an introduction to the science writing I have been doing online since 2008.

Addiction is a disease, although the precise definition of "disease" can and does vary greatly. It is a multi-faceted, complex condition, as the blog articles in this collection demonstrate. Addiction is commonly misunderstood, because it has prominent psychological symptoms and is strongly influenced by environment. Addiction isn't like cancer—although it is a good deal like diabetes, high blood pressure, and other chronic and potentially fatal disorders. Like these diseases, addiction does not diminish free will or personal responsibility in any way. If you have high blood pressure or diabetes, it is YOUR job to do something about it. And the same with addiction.

Articles need not be read in any particular order. Each post is followed by a link to its original onsite location, where a host of relevant links may be found.

The Research section includes posts on a wide-ranging and controversial group of subjects, all related by an approach that highlights the underlying science and evidence-based medicine pertinent to the subject. Is shoplifting the opiate of the masses? Does menthol really matter? Can ketamine and other party drugs cause permanent bladder damage? For answers, I look to neuroscientists and addiction researchers, an approach that led to my earlier book, *The Chemical Carousel: What Science Tells Us About Beating Addiction*. Science has also guided the work at Addiction Inbox since 2008.

The section on the New Synthetics fires a few shots at a moving target, in an effort to help readers keep up with what's happening in the scary new world of bath salts and spice. These drugs, and more like them, won't be going away overnight. They now must be added to the already bewildering mix of addictive drugs driving the worldwide drug trade—an industry too big to measure, as it busily builds entirely new chemicals under the sun.

In the section on Treatment, I have culled a variety of posts, far too many of which have to do with vital flaws in the treatment programs and paradigms offered to addicts in today's recovery bazaar. The disconnect between addiction science and the American for-profit treatment industry is addressed in this section. And finally, in a section devoted to Interviews and Book Reviews, I feature the words of prominent scientists, researchers, and addicts themselves. There is always room for good books and good conversation.

I thank Dr. Angela Browne-Miller for her invitation to contribute a chapter to the 2009 *Praeger International Collection on Addictions*.

Introduction

I also thank the College on Problems of Drug Dependence for the recognition and financial support that came my way as the recipient of its 2012 Media Award. And I would be remiss not to mention the valuable insights on blogging provided by the annual ScienceOnline conferences I have attended in North Carolina's Research Triangle.

Finally, I'd like to give credit to just a few of the many scientists and writers who are part of an informal coterie of online colleagues who lend some gravitas to the concept of online social media. I am attached to this band of thinkers and doers primarily through Twitter, which is not always about what somebody in pajamas had for lunch.

I thank Maia Szalavitz of Time Healthland, pharmacologist David Kroll at the North Carolina Museum of Natural Sciences, Forbes science blogger Emily Willingham, research psychologist Vaughan Bell at King's College in London, Daniel Lende at the University of South Florida's Department of Anthropology, Reuters Health Executive Editor Ivan Oransky, Sanho Tree of the Drug Policy Project, patient advocate blogger Laura Newman, addiction blogger Cassie Rodenberg, Robin Lloyd at Scientific American, science blogger Jason Goldman, neuroscience lecturer Jon Simons at the University of Cambridge, Nicky Penttila at the Dana Foundation, Michael Farrell of Australia's National Drug and Alcohol Research Center, neuropsychology professor Keith Laws at the University of Hertfordshire, Professor Howard Shaffer of Harvard Medical School, Michael Taffe at the Scripps Research Institute, novelist and professor Jim Brown at UC-San Bernardino, Deni Carise of Phoenix House, UCLA-trained addiction expert Dr. Adi Jaffe, neuroscience professor Marc Lewis at Radboud University in The Netherlands, the drug researcher who blogs as Drugmonkey, the postdoc who blogs as Scicurious, and, finally, Scientific American's Blog Editor—the Blogfather himself—Bora Zivkovic.

Table of Contents

Table of Contents

1) Research

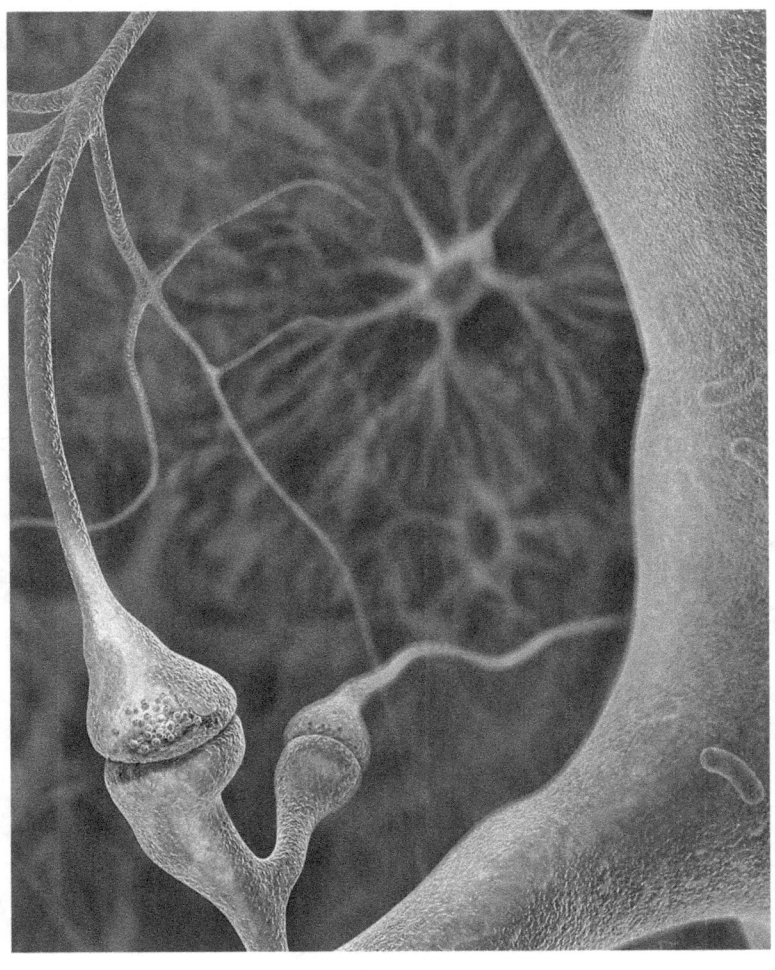

(National Institute of Drug Abuse)

Decoding Dope

Why marijuana gets you high, and hemp doesn't.

Cannabis sativa comes in two distinct flavors—smokeable weed, and headache-inducing hemp. The difference between hemp and smokeable marijuana is simple: Hemp, used for fiber and seed, contains only a tiny amount of THC, the primary active ingredient in the kind of cannabis that gets you high. I am old enough to recall the sad saga of California hippies driving through my natal state of Iowa, and filling their trunks with "ditch weed"—wild hemp that grows commonly along Iowa rural fencerows, and while it cannot get you high, it could, back then, get you arrested.

But the California hippies who ran afoul of the law in Iowa were not so stupid as it might seem. Even a marijuana connoisseur can have a hard time telling the difference between strong sinsemilla and wild hemp. Both varieties look similar, have similar growth patterns and flowering schedules, and a fresh bud of ditch hemp can look and smell enticingly like the real thing. Even the trichomes—the thousands of sticky, microscopic stalks that grow on the female flowers, each containing a bead of resin, like a crystal golf ball on a tee, containing mostly THC, in the case of pot, and mostly CBD, in the case of hemp—are also similar in appearance and growth behavior.

A study by a group of Canadian researchers, published in *Genome Biology*, lays out the draft genome of marijuana, containing all of

3

the plant's hereditary information as encoded in DNA and RNA. In their article, Timothy Hughes, Jonathan Page, and co-workers reported "a draft genome and transcriptome sequence of C. sativa Purple Kush." (The genome and transcriptome can be browsed or downloaded at The Cannabis Genome Browser.) **More than 20 plant genomes have now been sequenced, including corn and rice, but cannabis sativa marks the first genomic sequencing of a traditional medicinal plant.**

So how does it happen that one version of cannabis comes power packed, while the other version shoots blanks, so to speak? The researchers began with the modern facts of the matter: The THC content of medical and recreational marijuana is "remarkably high." Research shows that median levels of THC in dried female flowers of Purple Kush (the strain used in the study) and other high-end variants now approach 11%, with some strains achieving a stratospheric 23% THC content by dry weight. Why can't breeders pull any buzz out of ditch weed? How did cannabis split into two distinct subtypes? In an accompanying editorial entitled "how hemp got high," Naomi Attar calls cannabis sativa "a plant with a 'split personality,' whose Dr. Jekyll, hemp, is an innocent source of textiles, but whose Mr. Hyde, marijuana, is chiefly used to alter the mind." **In brief, what are the biological reasons for the psychoactive differences between marijuana and hemp?**

Co-lead author Jon Page, a plant biologist at the University of Saskatchewan, along with Tim Hughes of the Department of Molecular Genetics at the University of Toronto, compared the genomic information of Purple Kush, a medical marijuana favorite, with a Finnish strain of hemp called Finola, which was developed for oil seed production and contains less than 1% THC content. That is not enough THC to be mind-altering in any way. Instead, what Finola has in abundance is cannabidiol, or CBD, the other major ingredient in cannabis.

CBD isn't considered psychoactive, but it does produce a host of pharmacological activity in the body. CBD shows less affinity for the two main types of cannabis receptors, CB1 and CB2, meaning that it attaches to receptors more weakly, and activates them less robustly, than THC. **The euphoric effects of marijuana are generally attributed to THC content, not CBD content**. In fact, there appears to be an inverse ratio at work. According to a paper in *Neuropsychopharmacology*, "Delta-9-THC and CBD can have opposite effects on regional brain function, which may underlie their different symptomatic and behavioral effects, and CBD's ability to block the psychotogenic effects of delta-9-THC."

The kind of cannabis people want to buy has a high THC/low CBD profile, while the hemp chemotype is just the reverse—low THC/high CBD. **While the medical marijuana movement has concentrated on Purple Kush and other high-THC breeds, medical researchers have often tilted towards the CBD-heavy variants, since CBD seems to be directly involved with some of the purported medicinal effects of the plant.** So, CBD specifically does not produce the usual marijuana high with accompanying euphoria and forgetfulness and munchies. What other researchers have discovered is that pot smokers who suffer the most memory impairment are the ones smoking cannabis low in cannabidiol, while people smoking cannabis high in cannabidiol—cheap, seedy, brown weed—show almost no memory impairment at all. THC content didn't seem to matter. It was the percentage of CBD that controlled the degree of memory impairment, the authors of earlier studies concluded.

The researchers found evidence in Purple Kush for "upregulation of cannabinoid 'pathway genes' and the exclusive presence of functional THCA synthase." That means the reason hemp doesn't get you high is because it is lacking the crucial enzyme—THCA synthase—that limits production of CBD and allows the production of THC to go wild. In contrast, cannabis strains producing high levels of THC—the Kushes and Hazes and White Widows and other seriously spendy variants—*do* have high levels of the enzyme that limits the production of CBD. Purple Kush gets you high because it has a built-in chemical brake on the production of CBD. Hemp doesn't.

In a press release from the University of Saskatchewan, the researchers explain how they think this divergence came about: "Over thousands of years of cultivation, hemp farmers selectively bred Cannabis sativa into two distinct strains—one for fiber and seed, and one for medicine." This intensive selective breeding resulted in changes in the essential enzyme for THC production, which "is turned on in marijuana, but switched of in hemp," as Page put it. **Furthermore, says co-leader Tim Hughes of the Department of Molecular Genetics at the University of Toronto, an additional enzyme responsible for removing materials required for THC production was "highly expressed in the hemp strain, but not the Purple Kush."** The loss of this enzyme in Purple Kush eliminated a substance "which would otherwise compete for the metabolites used as starting material" in THC production.

Without knowing the mechanics of it, underground growers and breeders have been steadily maximizing the cultivation of strains of cannabis high in THCA synthase, the result of which is a molecular blocking maneuver that maximizes THC production. This is great for getting high, but may not be the optimal breeding strategy for producing plants with medicinal properties. Raphael Mechoulam, the scientist who first isolated and synthesized THC, has referred to plant-derived cannabinoids as a "neglected pharmacological treasure trove." The authors of this study agree, and have already identified some candidate genes that encode for a variety of cannabinoids with "interesting biological activities." Such knowledge, they say, will "facilitate breeding of cannabis for medical and pharmaceutical applications."

But cannabis of this kind may turn out to be low-THC weed. And that may be a good thing, some researchers believe. Marijuana expert Lester Grinspoon told *Nature News*: "Cannabis with high cannabidiol levels will make a more appealing option for anti-pain, anti-anxiety and anti-spasm treatments, because they can be delivered without causing disconcerting euphoria." (We'll leave definitional issues about the effects of euphoria for another post.)

Finally, the authors strongly suggest that if it were not for "legal restrictions in most jurisdictions on growing cannabis, even for research purposes," we would have known all of this stuff years ago, and would have been well on our way to developing "finer tailoring of cannabinoid content in new strains of marijuana," as *Nature News Blog* describes it.

Sunday, October 23, 2011

http://addiction-dirkh.blogspot.com/2011/10/decoding-dope.html

van Bakel H, Stout JM, Cote AG, Tallon CM, Sharpe AG, Hughes TR, & Page JE (2011). The draft genome and transcriptome of Cannabis sativa. *Genome biology, 12* (10) PMID: 22014239

The Biology of Stimulants, or Why You Can't Stay High Forever

An essay on the losing battle for perpetual reward.

The amphetamine high, like the cocaine high, is a marvel of biochemical efficiency. Stimulants work primarily by blocking the reuptake of dopamine molecules in the synaptic gap between nerve cells. Dopamine remains stalled in the gap, stimulating the receptors, resulting in higher dopamine concentrations and greater sensitivity to dopamine in general. Since dopamine is involved in moods and activities such as pleasure, alertness and movement, the primary results of using cocaine or speed—euphoria, a sense of well being, physical alertness, and increased energy—are easily understood. Even a layperson can tell when lab rats have been on a meth binge. The rapid movements, sniffing, and sudden rearing at minor stimuli are not that much different in principle from the outward signs of meth intoxication among higher primates.

Chemically, cocaine and amphetamine are very different compounds. Psychoactively, however, they are very much alike. Of all the addictive drugs, smoked cocaine and speed have the most direct and most devastatingly euphoric effect on the dopamine systems of the brain. Cocaine and amphetamine produce rapid classical conditioning in addicts, demonstrated by the intense cravings touched off by such stimuli as the sight of a building where the user used to buy or sell. Environmental impacts of this nature can produce marked blood flow increases to key limbic structures in abstinent addicts.

In clinical settings, cocaine users have a hard time distinguishing between equal doses of cocaine and Dexedrine, administered intravenously. As we know, it is the shape of the molecule that counts. The amphetamines are shaped like dopamine and norepinephrine, two of the three reward chemicals. Speed, then, is well suited to the task of artificially stimulating the limbic reward pathway. **Molecules of amphetamine displace dopamine and norepinephrine in the storage vesicles, squeezing those two neurotransmitters into the synaptic gap and keeping them there.** By mechanisms less well identified, cocaine accomplishes the same feat. Both drugs also interfere with the return of dopamine, norepinephrine, and serotonin molecules to their storage sacs, a procedure known as reuptake blocking. Cocaine works its effects primarily by blocking the reuptake of dopamine.

Amphetamine was once one of the most widely prescribed drugs in the pharmacological cornucopia. It exists in large part now as a recreational drug of choice, abuse, and addiction. The same is true of cocaine. It was replaced as a dental anesthetic long ago, in favor of non-addictive variants like Novocain. The same tragic list of statistical side effects that apply to abusers of alcohol, heroin and nicotine also apply to stimulant abusers: Increased risk of car accidents, homicides, heart attack, and strokes.

In the late 1990s, scientists at Johns Hopkins and NIDA showed that opiate receptors play a role in cocaine addiction as well. **PET scans demonstrated that cocaine addicts showed increased binding activity at mu opiate receptors sites in the brain during active cocaine addiction.** Take away the cocaine, and the brain must cope with too many empty dopamine and endorphin receptors. It is also easy to understand the typical symptoms of cocaine and amphetamine withdrawal: lethargy, depression, anger, and a heightened perception of pain. Both the cocaine high and the amphetamine high are easily augmented with cigarettes or heroin. **These combinations result in "nucleus accumbens dopamine overflow," a state of neurochemical super saturation similar to the results obtained with the notorious "speedball"—heroin plus cocaine.**

With the arrival of smokable forms of cocaine and amphetamine, the race to pin down the biology of stimulation became even more urgent. Stimulants in smokable form—crack and ice—are even more rapidly addictive for addiction-prone users. "The reason has to do with the hydraulics of the blood supply," a researcher at the University of Minnesota explained to me. **"High concentrations are achieved with each inhalation, and sent right upstairs to the brain—but not all of the brain simultaneously. The target of the flow of blood is the limbic system, whereas the remainder of the brain is exposed to much milder concentrations."**

This extraordinarily concentrated jolt to the reward center is the reason why smokable cocaine and speed are able to pack such a wallop. The entire range of stimulative effects hits the ventral tegmental area and associated reward regions of the brain in seconds, and the focused nature of the impact yields an astonishingly pleasurable high.

But the long-term result is exactly the opposite. It may sound dour and religious, but the scientific fact of the matter is that continuous chemical pleasure extracts its fee in the end: The body's natural stock of these neurotransmitters starts to fall as the brain, striving to compensate for the artificial flooding of the reward center, orders a general cutback in production. At the same time, the receptors for these neurotransmitters become excessively sensitive due to the frequent, often unremitting nature of the stimulation.

"It's clear that cocaine causes depletion of dopamine, norepinephrine, serotonin—it is a general neurotransmitter depleter," said my research source. "That may account for many of the effects we see after someone has stopped using cocaine. They're tired, they're lethargic, they sleep; they may be depressed, moody, and so on." **Continued abuse of stimulant drugs only makes the problem worse.** One reason why cocaine and amphetamine addicts will continue to use, even in the face of rapidly diminishing returns, is simply to avoid the crushing onset of withdrawal. Even though the drugs may no longer be working as well as they once did, the alternative—the psychological cost of withdrawal—is even worse. In the jargon used by Alcoholics Anonymous, addicts generally have to get worse before they can get better.

When addicts talk about "chasing a high," the metaphor can be extended to the losing battle of neurotransmitter levels.

Wednesday, September 28, 2011

http://addiction-dirkh.blogspot.com/2011/09/biology-of-stimulants-or-why-you-cant.html

Heroin in Vietnam: The Robins Study Reexamined

How everything we knew about heroin was wrong.

In 1971, under the direction of Dr. Jerome Jaffe of the Special Action Office on Drug Abuse Prevention, Dr. Lee Robins of Washington University in St. Louis undertook an investigation of heroin use among young American servicemen in Vietnam. Nothing about addiction research would ever be quite the same after the Robins study. **The results of the Robins investigation turned the official story of heroin completely upside down.**

The dirty secret that Robins laid bare was that a staggering number of Vietnam veterans were returning to the U.S. addicted to heroin and morphine. Sources were already reporting a huge trade in opium throughout the U.S. military in Southeast Asia, but it was all mostly rumor until Dr. Robins surveyed a representative sample of enlisted Army men who had left Vietnam in September of 1971—the date at which the U.S. Army began a policy of urine screening. The Robins team interviewed veterans within a year after their return, and again two years later.

After she had worked up the interviews, Dr. Robins, who died in 2009, found that almost half—45 per cent—had used either opium or heroin at least once during their tour of duty. 11 per cent had tested positive for opiates on the way out of Vietnam. **Overall, about 20 per cent reported that they had been addicted**

to heroin at some during their term of service. To put it in the kindest possible light, military brass had vastly underestimated the problem. One out of every five soldiers in Vietnam had logged some time as a junky. **As it turned out, soldiers under the age of 21 found it easier to score heroin than to hassle through the military's alcohol restrictions. The "gateway drug hypothesis" didn't seem to function overseas.** In the United States, the typical progression was assumed to be from "soft" drugs (alcohol, cigarettes, and marijuana) to the "hard" category of cocaine, amphetamine, and heroin. In Vietnam, soldiers who drank heavily almost never used heroin, and the people who used heroin only rarely drank. The mystery of the gateway drug was revealed to be mostly a matter of choice and availability. One way or another, addicts found their way to the gate, and pushed on through.

"Perhaps our most remarkable finding," Robins later noted, **"was that only 5% of the men who became addicted in Vietnam relapsed within 10 months after return, and only 12% relapsed even briefly within three years."** What accounted for this surprisingly high recovery rate from heroin, thought to be the most addictive drug of all? As is turned out, treatment and/or institutional rehabilitation didn't make the difference: Heroin addiction treatment was close to nonexistent in the 1970s, anyway. "Most Vietnam addicts were not even detoxified while in service, and only a tiny percentage were treated after return," Robins reported. It wasn't solely a matter of easier access, either, since roughly half of those addicted in Vietnam had tried smack at least once after returning home. But very few of them stayed permanently readdicted.

Any way you looked at it, too many soldiers had become addicted, many more than the military brass had predicted. But somehow, the bulk of addicted soldiers toughed their way through it, without formal intervention, after they got home. Most of them kicked the habit. Even the good news, then, took some getting used to. The Robins Study painted a picture of a majority of soldiers kicking it on their own, without formal intervention. For some of them, kicking wasn't even an issue. They could "chip" the drug at will—they could take it or leave it. And when they came home, they decided to leave it.

However, there was that other cohort, that 5 to 12 per cent of the servicemen in the study, for whom it did not go that way at all. This group of former users could not seem to shake it, except with great difficulty. And when they did, they had a very strong tendency to relapse. Frequently, they could not shake it at all, and rarely could they shake it for good and forever. Readers old enough to remember Vietnam may have seen them at one time or another over the years, on the streets of American cities large and small. Until quite recently, only very seriously addicted people who happened to conflict with the law ended up in non-voluntary treatment programs.

The Robins Study sparked an aggressive public relations debate in the military. Almost half of America's fighting men in Vietnam had evidently tried opium or heroin at least once, but if the Robins numbers were representative of the population at large, then relatively few people who tried opium or heroin faced any serious risk of long-term addiction. A relative small number of users were not so fortunate, as Robins noted. What was the difference?

Tuesday, January 24, 2012

http://addiction-dirkh.blogspot.com/2012/01/heroin-in-vietnam-robins-study.html

Robins, Lee N. (1994). "Lessons from the Vietnam Heroin Experience." Harvard Mental Health Letter. December.
See also: Robins, Lee. N. (1993) "Vietnam veterans' rapid recovery from heroin addiction: a fluke or normal expectation?" Addiction. 88(8), 1037 – 1167.

Cigarette Sadness

The chemistry of sorrow during nicotine withdrawal.

When you smoke a cigarette, nicotine pops into acetylcholine receptors in the brain, the adrenal glands, and the skeletal muscles, and you get a nicotine rush. Just like alcohol, a cigarette alters the transmission of several important chemical messengers in the brain. **"These are not trivial responses," said Professor Ovide Pomerleau of the University of Michigan Medical School. "It's like lighting a match in a gasoline factory."**

Experiments at NIDA's Addiction Research Center in Baltimore have confirmed that nicotine withdrawal not only makes people irritable, but also impairs intellectual performance. Logical reasoning and rapid decision-making both suffer during nicotine withdrawal. Acetylcholine appears to enhance memory, which may help explain a common lament voiced by many smokers during early withdrawal. **As summarized by one ex-smoker, "I cannot think, cannot remember, cannot concentrate."**

But there is another, less widely discussed aspect of nicotine withdrawal: profound sadness. Profound enough, in many cases, to be diagnosed as clinical unipolar depression.

Of course, people detoxing from addictive drugs like nicotine are rarely known to be happy campers. **But quitting smoking, for all its other withdrawal effects, reliably evokes a sense of acute nostalgia, like saying goodbye to a lifelong**

friend. The very act of abstinence produces sadness, joylessness, dysphoria, melancholia—all emotional states associated with unipolar depression.

Work undertaken by Dr. Alexander Glassman and his associates at the New York State Psychiatric Institute has nailed down an unexpectedly strong relationship between prior depression and cigarette smoking, and the findings have been confirmed in other work. This sheds important light on the question of why some smokers repeatedly fail to stop smoking, regardless of the method or the motivation. The problem, as Glassman sees it, is "an associated vulnerability between affective [mood] disorders and nicotine."

Now a group of Canadian researchers, working out of the Centre of Addiction and Mental Health (CAMH) and the Department of Psychiatry at the University of Toronto, believe they have isolated the specific neuronal mechanisms responsible for the profound sadness of the abstinent smoker.

Writing in the *Archives of General Psychiatry*, the investigators, who had access to what the CAMH proudly calls the only PET scanner in the world dedicated to mental health and addiction research, gave PET scans to 24 healthy smokers and 24 healthy non-smokers. Non-smokers were scanned once, while heavy and moderate cigarette smokers were scanned after smoking a cigarette, and also after a period of acute withdrawal. Earlier research of this kind had focused on nicotine's effect on dopamine release. **But Ingrid Bacher and her coworkers in Toronto were measuring MAO-A levels in the prefrontal and anterior cingulate regions, two areas known to be involved in "affect," or emotional responses**. When patients suffering from major depressive disorders get scanned, they tend to show elevated levels of MAO-A. The so-called MAO-A inhibitors Marplan, Nardil, Emsam, and Parnate are still in use as antidepressant medications. In general, the higher the levels of MAO-A, the lower the levels of various neurotransmitters crucial to pleasure and reward. A high level of MAO-A would suggest that the enzyme was significantly altering the activity of serotonin, dopamine, and norepinephrine in brain regions involved in mood.

The researchers found that smokers in withdrawal had 25-35% more MAO-A binding activity than non-smoking controls. "This finding may explain why heavy smokers are at high risk for clinical depression," says Dr. Anthony Phillips, Scientific Director of the Canadian Institutes of Health Research's (CIHR's) Institute of Neurosciences, Mental Health and Addiction, which funded this study.

Although researchers involved in these kinds of drug studies almost always claim that the work is likely to lead to new pharmacological therapies, the plain truth is that such immediate spinouts are rare. **But in this case, it does seem like the study provides a clear incentive to investigate the clinical standing of MAO-A inhibitors as an adjunct therapy in stop-smoking programs**. "Understanding sadness during cigarette withdrawal is important because this sad mood makes it hard for people to quit, especially in the first few days," said Dr. Jeffrey Meyer, one of the study authors.

As one addiction researcher noted, an associated vulnerability to depression "isn't going to cover everybody's problem, and it doesn't mean that if you give up smoking, you're automatically going to plunge into a suicidal depression. However, for people who have some problems along those lines, giving up smoking definitely complicates their lives."

Thursday, August 4, 2011

http://addiction-dirkh.blogspot.com/2011/08/cigarette-sadness.html

Bacher, I., Houle, S., Xu, X., Zawertailo, L., Soliman, A., Wilson, A., Selby, P., George, T., Sacher, J., Miler, L., Kish, S., Rusjan, P., &

Meyer, J. (2011). Monoamine Oxidase A Binding in the Prefrontal and Anterior Cingulate Cortices During Acute Withdrawal From Heavy Cigarette Smoking *Archives of General Psychiatry, 68* (8), 817-826 DOI: 10.1001/archgenpsychiatry.2011.82

Night Owls Get a Coffee Break

"Morning people" have more caffeine-related sleep problems.

Let me start by saying that I love this caffeine study for personal reasons. As a lifelong night owl, I have been chastised by wife, family, and friends over the years for my regular habit of drinking coffee after 10 pm. (And falling easily asleep two or three hours later, if I choose to.) Other coffee drinkers have told me how rare and weird this is. If we have a cup, they tell me, or even an afternoon sip, we toss and turn all night.

As it turns out, I was talking to the wrong kind of coffee drinkers. I needed to consult my crowd, and that's what I did. **I checked in with a few confirmed fellow night owls, and yes, a few of them reported that they had no problems going to sleep after a late night cup or two.**

Anecdotal, of course—but a recent clinical study published in *Sleep Medicine* backs me up. The study, "Modeling caffeine concentrations with the Stanford Caffeine Questionnaire: Preliminary evidence for an interaction of chronotype with the effects of caffeine on sleep," sets out to examine the effects of caffeine on the sleep patterns of college students. Researchers at Stanford told the students to keep sleep logs and to wear an actigraphy wristband to record rest/activity cycles. The students filled out daily questionnaires about their caffeine intake at different times of the day, and gave saliva samples for caffeine assessments.

The scientists were able to accurately predict salivary caffeine concentrations based on the questionnaires, which was the primary intent of the study. **But in the process, they discovered what they believe to be "a novel relationship between the effects of caffeine on sleep and genotype and chronotype."** What the researchers ended up with was some seriously suggestive evidence about the relationship of caffeine and natural sleep rhythms.

Typically, clinical trials with caffeine are limited to the basic question: How much coffee did you drink today? But the Stanford researchers wanted to include the many variables that modulate caffeine intake—things like the timing of ingestion, the variations in the amount of caffeine among beverages, individual variations in caffeine metabolism, and the wide differences in half-life that caffeine can exhibit under various circumstances. They attempted to establish the students' genotypes for adenosine receptors, where caffeine does most of its work, and to select volunteers who had "statistically indistinguishable" differences in adenosine receptor gene frequencies.

As you might expect, even among students, caffeine intake progressively decreased throughout the day in the study group. **However, a small number of participants continued their intake of caffeine well into the night.** The metric known as "wake after sleep onset," or WASO, was used as the primary measurement of sleep disruption. "Our data indicate caffeine strongly influences WASO in those who self-identify as morning-type," the researchers found. "It affects WASO less so in those who are neither type, and does not appear to affect WASO in those who are evening-type. To our knowledge, there have been no previous reports linking the effects of caffeine and chronotype."

Some warnings on the study: It involved only 50 college students. And they were *students*, meaning their schedules were highly erratic by definition, and they were chronically sleep-deprived by habit. The study authors attempted to turn this defect into a virtue, noting that "the students were under such homeostatic pressure that their mood had little effect on their sleep." Nonetheless, we will need to see if the findings hold up using less, er, unpredictable subjects.

If they *do* hold up, it will make it easier for people to understand the homily delivered by the coffee-drinking grandmother of a friend of mine: "The only time coffee ever kept me awake was when I knew there was another cup in the pot."

Sunday, March 4, 2012

http://addiction-dirkh.blogspot.com/2012/03/night-owls-get-coffee-break.html

Nova, P., Hernandez, B., Ptolemy, A., & Zeitzer, J. (2012). Modeling caffeine concentrations with the Stanford Caffeine Questionnaire: Preliminary evidence for an interaction of chronotype with the effects of caffeine on sleep *Sleep Medicine* DOI: 10.1016/j. sleep.2011.11.011

Energy Drinks: What's the Big Deal?

The sons of Red Bull are sporting record concentrations of caffeine.

Are energy drinks capable of pushing some people into caffeine-induced psychotic states? Some medical researchers think so, under the right set of conditions.

Red Bull, for all its iconic ferocity, is pretty tame, weighing in at approximately half a cup of coffee. Drinks like Monster Energy and Full Throttle push it up to 100-150 milligrams of caffeine, or the equivalent of a full cuppa joe, according to USDA figures. That doesn't sound so bad—unless you're ten years old. A little caffeine might put you on task, but an overdose can leave you scattered and anxious—or worse. If you cut your teeth on Coke and Pepsi, then two or three energy drinks can deliver an order-of-magnitude overdose by comparison.

Readers are entitled to ask: Are you serious? Can't we just ignore the inevitable view-this-with-alarm development in normal kid culture, and move on?

My interest began when I ran across a 2009 case report in *CNS Spectrums*, describing an apparent example of "caffeine-induced delusions and paranoia" in a very heavy coffee drinking farmer. "Convinced of a plot against him," the psychologists write, "he installed surveillance cameras in his house and on his farm.... He became so preoccupied with the alleged plot that he neglected the business of the farm.... and he had his children taken from him because of unsanitary living conditions."

The patient was not known to be a drinker, reporting less than a case of beer annually. He had shown no prior history of psychotic behaviors. But for the past seven years, he had been consuming about 36 cups of coffee per day, according to his account. Take that number of cups times 125 milligrams, let's say, for a daily total of 4500 milligrams. At that level, he should be suffering from panic and anxiety disorders, according to caffeine toxicity reports, and he would be advised to call the Poison Control Center. And that certainly seems to have been the case. **"At presentation," the authors write, "the patient reported drinking 1 gallon of coffee/day."**

On the one hand, the idea of caffeine causing a state resembling chronic psychosis is the stuff of sitcoms. On the other hand, metabolisms do vary, and the precise manner in which coffee stimulates adenosine receptors can lead to anxiety, aggression, agitation, and other conditions. Could caffeine, in an aberrant metabolism, break over into full-blown psychosis? At the Caffeine Web, where psychiatrists and toxicologists duke it out online over all things caffeinated, Sidney Kay of the Institute of Legal Medicine writes: **"Coffee overindulgence is overlooked many times because the bizarre symptoms may resemble and masquerade as an organic or mental disease."** Symptoms, he explains, can include "restlessness, silliness, elation, euphoria, confusion, disorientation, excitation, and even violent behavior with wild, manic screaming, kicking and biting, progressing to semi-stupor."

That doesn't sound so good. In "Energy drinks: What is all the hype?" Mandy Rath examines the question in a recent issue of the *Journal of the American Academy of Health Practitioners.*

Selling energy drinks to kids from 6 to 19 years old is a $3.5 billion annual industry, Rath asserts. And while "most energy drinks consumed in moderation do not pose a huge health risk," more and more youngsters are putting away higher and higher doses of caffeine. At the level of several cans of Coke, or a few cups of strong coffee or, an energy drink or three, students can expect to experience improved reaction times, increased aerobic endurance, and less sleepiness behind the wheel. Most people can handle up to 300 mg of caffeine in a concentrated blast. Certainly a better bargain, overall, than three or four beers.

But first of all, you don't need high-priced, caffeine-packed superdrinks to achieve that effect. A milligram of caffeine is a milligram of caffeine. But wait, what about the nifty additives in Full Throttle and Monster and Rockstar? The taurine and… stuff. Taurine is an amino acid found in lots of foods. Good for you in the abstract. **Manufacturers also commonly add sugar (excess calories), ginseng (at very low levels), and bitter orange (structurally similar to norepinephrine).** However, the truly interesting addition is guarana, a botanical product from South America. When guarana breaks down, it's principal byproduct is, yes, caffeine. Guarana seeds contain twice the caffeine found in coffee beans. Three to five grams of guarana provide 250 mg of caffeine. Energy drink manufacturers don't add that caffeine to the total on the label because—oh wait, that's right, because makers of energy drinks, unlike makers of soft drinks, don't have to print the amount of caffeine as dietary information. **And on an ounce-for-pound basis, kids are getting a lot more caffeine with the new drinks than the older, labeled ones.**

All of this increases the chances of caffeine intoxication. Rath writes that researchers have identified caffeine-related increases among children in hypertension, insomnia, motor tics, irritability, and headaches. Chronic caffeine intoxication results in "anxiety, emotional disturbances, and chronic abdominal pain." Not to mention cardiac arrhythmia, seizures, and mania.

So what have we learned, kids? Energy drinks are safe—if you don't guzzle several of them in a row, or substitute them for dinner, or have diabetes, or an ulcer, or happen to be pregnant, or are suffering from heart disease or hypertension. And if you do OD on high-caffeine drinks, it will not be pleasant: Severe palpitations, panic, mania, muscle spasms, etc. Somebody might even want to take you to the emergency room. Coaches and teachers need to keep a better eye out for caffeine intoxication.

Note: There is a "caffeine calculator" available at the Caffeine Awareness website, designed to determine whether you are a coffee addict. I can by no means swear to its scientific accuracy, but, based on my own, distinctly non-young person daily intake, the test told me that my consumption was likely to manifest itself as "high irritability, moodiness & personality disorders." Can I blame it all on those endless cokes we had as kids? Growing up in the Baby Boom suburbs, we all drank carbonated caffeine beverages instead of water. Nothing much has changed except the caffeine levels.

Sunday, May 20, 2012

http://addiction-dirkh.blogspot.com/2012/05/energy-drinks-whats-big-deal.html

Rath, M. Energy drinks: What is all the hype? The dangers of energy drink consumption *Journal of the American Academy of Nurse Practitioners, 24* (2), 70-76. 2012. DOI: 10.1111/j.1745-7599.2011.00689.x

Codeine Blues: End of the Line for an Opiate with Issues?

Canada, UK consider phasing out the drug.

Among the many memorable anecdotes that have been uttered at the opening of an AA or NA meeting, surely one of the great ones is this: "I'm an addict, and a heroin junky. I went to the dentist today, and he sent me home with a prescription for Tylenol 3. And I thought: Do I really want to endanger my sobriety over a shitty buzz like codeine?"

Canada and the United Kingdom are ready to phase it out entirely. The U.S. Food and Drug Administration (FDA) issued a warning about it for nursing mothers as far back as 2007. Codeine, widely popular for its low euphoriant effects, and subsequent (if theoretical) decreased potential for abuse, may not be as strong as morphine and dilaudid, but it is perhaps the most commonly prescribed opiate in the world—and it comes with a major flaw. **Unlike other opiates, codeine is very unpredictable in its interactions with an enzyme called CYP2D6.** This enzyme is a primary workhorse in the body's process of breaking down and excreting many different drugs. Poor metabolizers produce less of this crucial enzyme, which means that drugs are broken down and excreted at a much slower pace.

Specifically, as two physicians recently wrote in the *Canadian Medical Association Journal*, "polymorphisms occur in the cytochrome

P450 isoenzyme CYP2D6 that enhance codeine metabolism to morphine." **In 2007, following the death of an infant nursed by a codeine-using mother, the FDA "warned nursing mothers that if they took codeine after childbirth, their newborns might be at risk for a morphine overdose," according to a *New York Times* report.**

Alternatively, other metabolizers may have little or no reaction to codeine-based medications. Drugs of abuse severely complicate these enzymatic issues, since addicts and alcoholics are not known for volunteering information about their condition to medical or hospital personnel.

Testing for the enzyme is possible, but not likely to catch on with cash-strapped medical and dental centers. Dr. Noni MacDonald at the University of Halifax and Dr. Stuart MacLeod at the University of British Columbia argue in the CMAJ that these genetic variations "can have potentially serious clinical consequences. **The wrong combination can result in toxic levels of morphine, even at conventional doses of codeine." The younger the user, the more susceptible he or she will be to these effects, "possibly because of age-related maturation differences in the blood-brain barrier."** The authors warned that serious side effects, "including life-threatening respiratory depression," have also been reported in adults.

The ultrafast metabolizing variant of CYP2D6 is not evenly distributed throughout the world's population. The number of people in danger of experiencing high morphine levels after codeine use range from 40% in North Africa to 3% in Europe, the authors say. Rates in the U.S. are 8%, meaning roughly one in ten Americans risk an adverse reaction when taking codeine.

Since the groups at highest risk are infants and children, nations have taken various steps to mitigate the risk. **"Switzerland sets the minimum age for codeine-based treatment at 1- years,**

the Netherlands at 1 year, the United States at 3 years and Canada at 2 years."

Despite these controls, the authors strongly argue for "a more direct approach," calling for doctors to "stop using the prodrug codeine altogether and instead use its active metabolite, morphine. Not only is the metabolism of morphine more predictable that that of codeine, but also it's cheaper." So codeine is just not consistently good at what it does. Problem is, an opiate doesn't have to be good to be great, as innumerable codeine addicts can attest.

The argument in Canada made sense to Britain's watchdog agency for medicines, the Medicines and Healthcare Products Regulatory Agency (MHRA). According to a report in *The Independent* by science editor Steve Connor, the MHRA "wrote to medical authorities in the UK warning that its experts have advised that all over-the-counter liquid cough medicines containing codeine should no longer be used in children under the age of 18," and that "the risks of [over-the-counter] cough medicines for children containing codeine outweigh the possible benefits."

Codeine is typically offered in paired form, with either acetaminophen or aspirin, as protection against opiate abuse. In theory, a drug abuser would be likely to trigger a Tylenol overdose before reaching an opiate overdose on codeine pills. However, it is perfectly possible to maintain an active opiate addiction on prescription Tylenol 3s, Fiorinal, or Phenergan cough syrup, among other drugs.

And finally, I would not be revealing any great secrets by suggesting that the extraction of codeine from a codeine-acetaminophen tablet through basic solubility and filtration procedures may not be something one needs to be a chemistry major to pull off.

The OTC medicine industry in the UK views all of this as a tired argument. A spokesperson for Britain's Proprietary Association, which represents over-the-counter manufacturers, said: "There has already been a long-drawn-out discussion of codeine. If its value as a pain reliever had not outweighed the risks then it would have been withdrawn and the point is that codeine still has a value as a pain reliever."

Sunday, October 17, 2010

http://addiction-dirkh.blogspot.com/2010/10/codeine-blues-
end-of-line-for-opiate.html

Sex, Drugs, and Sex

Pharmaceuticals and sexual performance.

The search for aphrodisiacs is an ancient, if not always venerable, human pursuit. Named for Aphrodite, the Greek goddess of love, aphrodisiacs are compounds that have the reputation, real or imagined, of increasing sexual desire, pleasure, and potency. It's safe to say that rhinoceros horn or tiger penis—various forms of sympathetic magic—just don't reliably do the trick.

Writing in *Hormones and Behavior*, a group of Canadian behavioral neurobiologists recently concluded that "substantial clinical and epidemiological literatures suggest that [stimulants and depressants] either inhibit sexual responding or can be 'prosexual' in certain situations, thereby increasing the potential of risky sexual activity and the spread of sexually transmitted diseases."

In other words, recreational drugs either sex you up, or they decrease your sex drive. And they either do or do not lead to risky sexual behavior among young people.

Not too promising a start. Nonetheless, JG Pfaus and coworkers at Concordia University's Center for Studies in Behavioral Neurobiology examined more than 100 studies based on animal models, and teased out some commonalities:

Stimulants are, well, stimulating. **Cocaine "facilitated penile erection" in male rats, while acute caffeine consumption amped up the sexual behavior of both male and female test animals.** As for depressants, small amounts of alcohol decreased inhibitory tendencies in rats, while a high level "disrupted sexual performance." Alcohol "increases rodent sexual motivation" but impairs specific parameters of sexual performance.

Yes, well, Shakespeare said it best. Macbeth proclaims at one point that alcohol "provokes the desire but it takes away the performance." As with mice, so with men and women. In animal studies, low doses of alcohol increase sexual desire, moderate doses intensify those effects, and a high dose extinguishes the impulse altogether. Male rodents, too, are subject to Brewer's Droop.

With the opiates, the story is much the same. In a National Institute on Drug Abuse (NIDA) study, the title of which— "Methadone reduces sexual performance and sexual motivation in the male Syrian golden hamster"—remains a classic, researchers found that after a dose of methadone, the critters were definitely disinclined to copulate. In general, systemic morphine inhibits sexual behavior in rats, mice, dogs, even donkeys. **Animals don't want to do it on opiates. Females stop engaging in "proceptive pacing and solicitation."**

And naturally, you're wondering about the sex lives of castrated Japanese quail. Researchers managed to get them copulating again with the opioid antagonist naloxone. (Testosterone implants also work.)

Although it sometimes seems laughable, there is a good argument to be made for the use of animals for modeling certain aspects of human sexual behavior. Stripped of cultural and complex social overlays, animal studies afford an opportunity to focus relentlessly on the biological. But enough for now on the fascinating topic of rats having sex on drugs.

In studies of men and women, Pfaus found that alcohol "dose-dependently delayed ejaculation, reduced the intensity of orgasm, and decreased both physiological and subjective measures of sexual arousal. Nearly identical effects were observed in women, although alcohol increased, rather than decreased, their subjective levels of sexual arousal." **The nastiest example of alcohol's effect on sex may be the blood vessel and nerve damage, sometimes permanent, known as chronic alcohol impotence**. Alcohol damage can disrupt communication between the pituitary gland and the genitals—and that can't be a good thing. Heavy smoking also reduces circulation to the blood vessels in the genitals. Heavy smokers and drinkers often report impotence or continuing sexually disinterest even when they have been sober and smokeless for a while.

Alcohol's effect on sexual performance is no secret, of course. But Pfaus also concludes that, in general, "drug use debilitates sexual responding in the majority of situations."

He means the whole pantheon, the entire roster of usual suspects: Why would drugs like cocaine, marijuana, amphetamine and oxycontin all have an overall negative effect on sexuality? Do hashish and cocaine, common "love potions" found in classical literature, boost sexual ardor, or do they have the opposite effect?

The following is a mix of anecdotal data and clinical reporting related to common addictive drugs and other "drugs of abuse."

LSD/Magic Mushrooms/Ecstasy/other Psychedelics: Some users report increased sexual awareness and sensitivity, but heavier doses tend to discourage sexual activity.

Marijuana/Hashish: Heightened sensory experiences can enhance sexual experiences, while heavier cannabis use can lower libido.

Cocaine: Equivocal. Users often report increased arousal and ease of orgasm. However, exactly the opposite effect is known to occur in heavy regular users.

Heroin/Oxycontin/other Opiates: Lowered libido and difficulty achieving orgasm are the norms. Yet even in this rather clear-cut case, there is no unanimity of opinion or experience. The familiar pattern is in evidence—a little bit might temporarily add some oomph to your sex drive. Heavier use is likely to lay a thick blanket across your libido.

Heroin is a strange case: In a 2003 study of women in methadone maintenance treatment programs, published in *Addictive Behaviors,* several different themes emerged: "Some women believe that drugs, particularly heroin, increase their sexual performance, libido, and pleasure, but for others, drugs, particularly crack cocaine, inhibit their sexual performance and desire. Many of the women believe that crack cocaine and heroin enhance a man's sexual desire, performance, and pleasure. However, other women deem that these drugs are responsible for their partner's abusive and coercive behavior." The effect of drugs on rates of sexual violence varies. Differential effects can be found in every aspect of the effect of drugs on sexual behavior, for the same reason that individuals vary in their response to these drugs. Metabolisms are not all the same.

Amphetamine: The stimulant rush can amp up sexual encounters; heavy use leads to desensitization and difficulty achieving orgasm. Intense but sometimes rather psychologically detached sex sessions can lead to everything from genital chafing to the classic "fuck knot" of tangled hair sometimes produced by a prolonged bout of missionary-position intercourse.

If the usual roster of recreational drugs cannot be counted on to perform as aphrodisiacs, there are always efforts underway to identify "prosexual" drugs and natural sex-enhancing nutrients. Among the contenders:

Bromocriptine (Parlodel): This drug is used to treat pituitary tumors and Parkinson's disease. It reduces prolactin, which is associated with age-related impotency in men. However, the dosage level required for the effect can cause unpleasant side effects.

Gamma-hydroxybutyrate (GHB): This one has been abused in the U.S. for its euphoric, sedative, and anabolic (body building) effects. It triggers the release of growth hormone from the pituitary. Not recommended. Combining GHB with alcohol sometimes leads to nausea and breathing problems.

DHEA: Big hopes were recently riding on this hormone. Sorry to say, Pfaus reports that in aging males, DHEA "had only transient effects in a well-controlled, double-blind study." Women had some promising hormonal news in the early going: "Mixed estrogen/androgen replacement to postmenopausal women improved measures of sexual desire, satisfaction, and frequency of sexual activity, compared with treatment with estrogen alone."

Yohimbe: Operating on a different receptor, this plant drug, long considered an aphrodisiac, pulls norepinephrine into the picture, at least in men. Yohimbine is an adrenoceptor agonist that fairly reliably turns on male rat mounting behavior and is reputed to be an effective sexual enhancer for some men.

Deprenyl (Seliginine): A dopamine booster, which also acts as a weird MAO inhibitor and is used for Parkinson's and depression, l-deprenyl has a reputation as a so-called smart drug, and is popular with life extension enthusiasts. It also markedly improves the sex lives of older rats. Another one with side effects to beware of.

There are also reports that L-dopa, used in patients with Parkinson's disease, increases sexual interest in the elderly. (But L-dopa has a number of undesirable side effects, too.) Apomorphine, a dopamine receptor agonist, increases the "likelihood of spontaneous erections."

In animal models, a variety of dopamine-active drugs generally have positive effects on the sexual behavior of rodents. As might be expected, drugs that block or reduce dopamine transmission also reduce sexual displays in animals. Our friend Drosophila melanogaster, the common fruit fly, doesn't get in the mood when it is dopamine-depleted, a state that can be reversed with L-dopa. Give a virgin male rat a good dose of D-amphetamine and it is off to the races, its surge of sexual excitement cause by dopamine release in the nucleus accumbens. In women, "the ability of estrogen to stimulate dopamine release and to augment dopamine release and behavior in response to amphetamine has been well established," according to James G. Pfaus and Barry J. Everitt in *The Psychopharmacology of Sexual Behavior*. But the specific mechanism by which this happens has not been identified.

Other scientists have also managed to sexually stimulate rats with extracts of *Turmera diffusa* (Damina), *Pfaffia paniculata* (Brazilian ginseng), and *Eurycoma longfolia Jak* (Catuaba).

As for serotonin, Pfaus and Everitt find "minimal methodologically-sound evidence on the effects on human sexuality of manipulating the serotoninergic system." So serotonin appears not to have much to do with sexual activity directly. In fact, it can have a negative effect, as users of SSRI antidepressants like Prozac have discovered. The common symptom in this case is difficulty achieving orgasm. Serotonin at 5-HT receptors inhibits sexual impulses in women as well as men.

In the end, Pfaus maintains that the best way to get male rats back in action after a strenuous day of copulation is "a combination of the nonspecific dopamine receptor agonist apomorphine and the adrenergic receptor antagonist yohimbine."

Thursday, July 28, 2011

http://addiction-dirkh.blogspot.com/2010/09/sex-drugs-and-sex.html

Pfaus, J., Wilkins, M., DiPietro, N., Benibgui, M., Toledano, R., Rowe, A., & Couch, M. (2010). Inhibitory and disinhibitory effects of psychomotor stimulants and depressants on the sexual behavior of male and female rats Hormones and Behavior, 58 (1), 163-176 DOI: 10.1016/j.yhbeh.2009.10.004.

Marijuana, Vomiting, and Hot Baths

A case history of cannabinoid hyperemesis.

Cannabinoid hyperemesis, as it's known, is an extremely rare but terrifying disorder marked by severe episodic vomiting that can only be relieved by hot baths. Sufferers are heavy, regular cannabis users, most of them. And hot baths? Where did THAT come from?

The syndrome was first brought to wider attention last year by the anonymous biomedical researcher known as Drugmonkey, **who documented cases of hyperemesis that had been reported in Australia and New Zealand, as well as Omaha and Boston in the U.S.** "There were two striking similarities across all these cases," Drugmonkey reported. "The first is that patients had discovered on their own that taking a hot bath or shower alleviated their symptoms. So afflicted individuals were taking multiple hot showers or baths per day to obtain symptom relief. The second similarity is, as you will have guessed, they were all cannabis users."

The reports haven't stopped. This summer, an intriguing account appeared on the official blog of New York University's Division of General Internal Medicine, where med students offered a formal definition: "A clinical syndrome characterized by intractable vomiting and abdominal pain associated with the unusual learned behavior of compulsive hot water bathing, occurring in the setting of long-term heavy marijuana use."

Still skeptical? I received this heartfelt comment on my original post a few days ago:

Listen, doubters. My son has this. He has been cyclical vomiting and spending hours in boiling hot baths since last Autumn. It's getting worse and he has lost a hell of a lot of weight. He is 21 and an addicted, heavy cannabis user who started at 15. He has tried cutting down but every other joint of weed brings on the obsession. He refuses to co operate with medical staff who try to treat him.

He has been taken to numerous hospitals as an emergency for non-stop vomiting and begs medical staff to let him sit in a very hot bath. They try the best anti-vomiting drugs instead, to no effect, and then some let him go in a hot shower for an hour plus. He always ends up on a drip and as soon as he feels well enough, discharges himself, often the same day.

At the weekend he went to a sports event in the city with friends, realised on the way he was going to have an episode, so left friends and made his way into a hotel room and locked himself in. Police were called and got him out of a boiling hot bath against his will. Cue vomiting attack so bad police called an ambulance. Once again discharged himself from hospital, demanding drip be removed or he would do it himself. Has sat in bath at house he shares with girlfriend for at least 12 hours today, she tells me. She says water is so hot she has no idea how he bears it.

He says he has no pain in stomach, just a sensation that drives his head mad and he KNOWS it will not go, or the vomiting stop, until he gets in boiling hot bath and stays there. He has even done this while abroad on holiday and ended up on a drip before being flown home.

All of this is true. A mother.

I was intrigued, and discussed this briefly with the mother, who lives in the U.K. She added a number of details in an email exchange, and agreed to let me publish her comments:

I am a mother in the UK whose son definitely has this, but is not officially diagnosed as he 'escapes' medical attention by discharging himself from various hospitals.

When it happens he is desperate to get in a hot bath. He lives with his girlfriend. I only realised what the hell was really going on when she insisted on telling me, and have since been regularly involved in the hospitals saga.

When I discovered the truth I put 'cannabis' 'vomiting' and 'hot baths' 'showers' in google and up came a perfect description of what my son does.

I am trying to get him to agree to go for counselling and psychiatric help as he has reached the stage where this obsessive vomiting and bathing is wrecking his life. But every time he gets a little better he believes he can 'control it' which is not the case at all.

Yes — we end up in the hospitals and the first young emergency doctor who has ever smoked a joint and/or thinks he knows everything, tells G "Oh no it can't be that, cannabis stops vomiting, not starts it." Of course, they have never heard of this condition and just think he is being irrational because of the constant need to vomit. They are sure it is food poisoning or some kind of spasm and take basic blood tests.

They find nothing, insist on giving him the best anti-sickness drugs usually for cancer patients and so on..., saying "this will definitely stop it" and still he vomits. He is not in pain, just rapidly dehydrating and panicking and complaining of a weird sensation in his stomach. He tells them "I know it's in my head doing this" and desperately demands to get in a bath. Even when he has arrived at hospital because police found him in a boiling hot bath, this makes no sense to the medics who only give in when none of their drugs work. He then immediately stops vomiting but is petrified of getting out of the bath. Eventually, when he says it is under control, he agrees to get out, and is put on a drip. Approx an hour later, while the doctors are planning follow-up procedures like scans and more complex blood tests etc, he starts an argument with a nurse, insists the drip is removed and phones a friend to collect him, avoiding seeking a lift from me if he can. The over-pressed doctors here (the British system is like a cattle market) are left mystified and move onto the next emergency in their pile up of admissions. And so it goes on, and will do, until G accepts even the odd joint can set him off.

- - - -

Researchers speculate that it has something to do with CB-1 cannabinoid receptors in the intestinal nerve plexus—but nobody really knows for sure. Low doses of THC might be anti-emetic, whereas in certain people, the high concentrations produced by long-term use could have the opposite effect.

Thursday, April 7, 2011

http://addiction-dirkh.blogspot.com/2011/04/marijuana-vomiting-and-hot-baths.html

Is Shoplifting the Opiate of the Masses?

Another look at "behavioral addictions" and the DSM-V.

The DSM-V, when it debuts, is set to replace the category of "Substance-Related Disorders" with a new category entitled "Addiction and Related Disorders." Gambling is the only behavioral addiction currently recommended for inclusion, but some experts have set their sights on shoplifting—an activity that is even more difficult to picture as a legitimate addiction than gambling. Or is it?

Long before gambling was widely looked upon as an addictive disorder, compulsive shoplifting already had a name: kleptomania. The National Association for Shoplifting Prevention claims that about 9-10% of the population show a "lifetime prevalence" for shoplifting. This is remarkably similar to the percentages commonly bandied about for alcoholics, drug addicts, unipolar depressives, compulsive gamblers, and compulsive overeaters.

A recent University of Florida survey pegged shoplifting losses, or "shrink," in 2009 at more than $11 billion annually. Plato, in *The Republic*, wanted to know whether thieves are made or born. It's a good question. Curiously, the stealing doesn't seem to be about money: The most recent study measuring income and shoplifting shows that Americans with incomes over $70,000 shoplift 30% more more than their fellow citizens earning less than $20,000 a year. And the actual items stolen by compulsive shoplifters often seem nonsensical, or even surreal. As director John Waters said of Pink Flamingos' star and compulsive shoplifter Divine: "I saw him walk out of a store once with a chain saw and a TV."

There is a definite "rush" to the act of stealing, writes Rachel Shteir in *The Steal*, her informative book about shoplifting. **One shoplifter said it was equal to drugs but only lasted a few minutes—"And you're back to yourself again. In your mind, you think, It was all for a stupid blouse, or stupid soap. For this, I risked everything."** Another source quoted in the book says, "I shoplifted every day, like someone with a drug addiction." Seconds before another women is arrested, she quizzes herself: "All she needs in the world is one crummy formal dress so why is there a blue silk jacket, one that she doesn't particularly like, in her camera bag?" And a shoplifting Lee Grant says in the movie "Detective Story": "I didn't need it. I didn't even like it." The objects seem to lose their intrinsic value once they have been stolen, and the shoplifter must get high again with another theft.

If, as some neurobiological researchers insist, addictive disorders are not independent disorders, but outward manifestations of an underlying disease pathology called addiction syndrome, then the definition might be stretched to include gambling, shoplifting, and certain other "activity-based expressions of addiction." Sometimes the alcoholic, the drug addict, the depressive, the compulsive gambler, and the obsessive overeater are all one and the same person. And drug addicts show a remarkably ability to substitute one drug for another. Perhaps a recovering cocaine addict might hope to assuage that sense of craving, of inchoate need, through excessive gambling. Or a shoplifter might use alcohol as a means of dampening the impulse to steal compulsively. While we don't use the term kleptomania anymore, "shoplifting crops up as a symptom of many types of mental illnesses—bipolar disorders and anxiety disorders as well as substance abuse, eating disorders, and depression," writes

Shteir. Compulsive shoplifting, Shteir concludes, is "as difficult to stamp out as oil spills or alcoholism."

For some, shoplifting brings a rush "similar to a cocaine or heroin high," according to psychiatist Jon Grant at the University of Minnesota School of Medicine. To find out just how similar, psychiatrists there tried treating shop-lifters with naltrexone, a drug that blocks opioid receptors and is used to treat alcoholism and heroin addiction. In 2009, in an article for the April issue of *Biological Psychiatry*, Grant and colleagues at the University of Minnesota School of Medicine recorded the results of their work with 25 kleptomaniacs, most of them women. All of the participants had been arrested for shoplifting at least once, and spent at least one hour per week stealing. The 8-week study is believed to be the first placebo-controlled trial of a drug for the treatment of shoplifting. In the April 10 issue of *Science*, Grant said that "Two-thirds of those on naltrexone had complete remission of their symptoms."

Thursday, September 1, 2011

http://addiction-dirkh.blogspot.com/2011/09/
is-shoplifting-opiate-of-masses.html

That Pesky Gambling Question

The DSM-V is set to label problem gambling an addiction

Nobody has ever bet enough on the winning horse.

—— Unknown wise person

I used to gamble. Back when I did, I was also an active alcoholic and a chain smoker. Camel filters, if you're wondering. And we had a running joke, my wife and I, although the humor leaked out of it for her pretty quickly. We would breach the doors of the gambling palace, and plunge into the dark, icy interior of a casino at Las Vegas or Tahoe, and stand on the edge of the gaming room, taking it all in for a moment. "Ah," I would say, surveying the roomful of cigarette smokers with drinks in their hands, making bets or hitting buttons at one o'clock in the morning, "my kind of people."

Gambling can be defined as an activity in which something of value is put at risk in a situation where the outcome is uncertain. That's really all there is to it. Howard J. Shaffer and Ryan Martin, whose article in the *Annual Review of Clinical Psychology*, "Disordered Gambling: Etiology, Trajectory and Clinical Considerations," takes on all the interesting questions about gambling as an addictive disease, have chosen to favor the term "disordered gambling." Just as there are divisions between alcoholic drinking, heavy drinking, and social drinking, there are similar states we can call pathological gambling, excessive gambling, and social gambling. **On the problematic end of the scale, pathological or problem gambling has proven to be "a more complex and unstable**

47

disorder than originally and traditionally thought." No kidding. Once the neurophysiology of the gambling state of mind came under scrutiny, the parallels with addiction cropped up so rapidly that investigators have been hard pressed to come up with suitable explanations for it all.

The new DSM-V proposes to shift pathological gambling from "impulse control disorder" to the new category of "addiction and related disorders." So it's a good time to rethink the question along with the psychiatric community.

In the traditional view, pathological gambling was a matter of exposure to the proper stimuli—it could happen to anyone. But as more and more gambling outlets and opportunities bloomed in Nevada, on reservations and riverboats, and in convenience stores, that view began to fall out of favor, because a funny thing happened. According to Shaffer and Martin, the prevalence of pathological gambling has remained stable over the past 35 years, even as opportunities to gamble have exploded. **The lifetime prevalence rate of pathological gambling in the U.S. in the mid-1970s was 0.7%, say the authors, and by 2005, U.S. lifetime rates had actually fallen slightly, to 0.6% or less. Where was the concomitant explosion in the number of pathological gamblers?**

Next, researchers got technical, wondering whether certain types of gambling, or certain types of gambling machines, were more "addictive" than others. They quickly ran into the same kind of trouble substance abuse researchers got into when they first tried ranking drugs according to strict hierarchies of addictiveness. In so doing, the staggering metabolic diversity of the human animal got lost in the shuffle, as did the fact that my metabolism and my behavior when taking drugs, or knocking one back, or losing money in a casino, is going to be different from yours.

Then came Internet gambling. **In 1996, the first online casino to accept real money began operation, and by 2001, there were more than a thousand.** Previously, researchers had to rely mostly on the time-honored but not always accurate system of self-reporting. If you ask people why they gamble, they tend to answer that they do it for the fun, the excitement, the challenge, and the chance to win some money. But what gamblers can't recall very well are specific patterns of play over time that might benefit researchers. For example, in a 2009 study in which observers actually watched gamblers gambling, one long-standing observation from the self-report literature—gamblers become more liberal risk takers as they approach the end of a gambling session in a behavior called "chasing"—didn't prove out. When researchers watched actual gamblers in action on the Internet, or playing lotteries, they found that problem gamblers in fact began betting more conservatively as they approached the end of their gambling, the authors write.

Another approach is to consider risk factors of all kinds—neurobiological, psychological, and social—and look for similarities between those for substance addiction, and those for "activity-based expressions of addiction." The "syndrome model," or what I usually call the umbrella model, derives from neurobiological research suggesting that "addictive disorders might not be independent: each outwardly unique addiction disorder might be a distinctive expression of the same underlying addiction syndrome.... The specific objects of addiction play a less central role in the development of addiction than previously thought...."

All of this opens the door to some informed speculation about a broader range of disorders that may lurk beneath the umbrella of the addictive disease concept. Among these are such conditions as body dysmorphic disorder, bulimia, depression, and extreme PMS, which are all found more often in addict populations. In addition, impulsivity and low "harm avoidance" are behavioral traits often found in association with addiction. Shaffer and Martin call these "shadow syndromes," and they are found to be associated with *both* substance and behavioral addictions.

But what, exactly, is the high in gambling? The researchers believe that, "similar to ingesting stimulants, there is evidence that gambling is associated with autonomic arousal including elevated blood pressure, heart rate, and mood." That's not very specific, and could also describe a craving for teddy bears. **But recently, fascinating evidence of neurobiological influences on gambling arose when Parkinson's' patients on strong dopamine agonist treatments, with no history of gambling whatsoever, began behaving for all the world like pathological gamblers.** I cannot imagine a better suggestion of neurogenetic involvement than this unexpected finding. Previous research had shown that dopamine-active drugs were capable of increasing the incidence of other addictions, too. Shaffer and Martin list compulsive eating, compulsive sexual behaviors, and compulsive shopping as activities that can also be boosted with dopamine agonists or diminished by lowering dopamine activity.

And it does not strike me as surprising to learn that, yes, gambling problems tend to run in families, or that twins studies show that pathological gambling is higher among twins born to pathological gamblers than twins born to non-gamblers. It is the same evidence anyone can bring forth to bolster the argument for neurobiological influences on alcoholism, heroin addiction, and the like. **"In sum" Shaffer and Martin conclude, "genetic influences might not determine the development of specific expression of addiction; however, genetics does influence the risk of addiction in general."**

If all of this is true, we should expect to see a corresponding connection between pathological gambling and substance abuse disorders. Some degree of overlap would be good evidence. And we have it in spades. **Pathological gamblers are five and a half times more likely to have suffered from a substance abuse disorder.** "75% of PGs (pathological gamblers) have had an alcohol disorder, 38% have had a drug use disorder and 60% have had nicotine dependence." Also, "PGs are 4 times more likely than non-PGs to experience a mood disorder in their lifetime...."

So when I used to stand on the edge of the casino floor, as an alcoholic and a nicotine addict, casually calling those gamblers my kind of people, I think I was more right than I ever could have guessed.

Does all this mean that playing games on the Internet is an addictive behavior if making bets with real money is involved? The authors crunched the studies on that question, and discovered that maybe 1% of the Internet population has used the Internet for gambling purposes, and that "the case of Internet gambling provides little evidence that exposure is the primary driving force behind the prevalence and intensity of gambling.... The relationship between the extent of gambling 'involvement' is a better predictor of disordered gambling than any particular game that people play."

By gambling involvement, the authors mean the number of different kinds of games a gambler plays. The more he or she plays, the more likely they are, or are likely to become, problem gamblers. However, it's not hard to see where the online notion came from. **Gambling folklore has always held that addiction is more of a risk with electronic gambling devices like slot machines and 5-Card Draw machines, than with traditional table games like roulette and craps.** But the authors don't find any convincing clinical evidence for this assertion at all. Internet gambling isn't more addictive, and doesn't confer any extra risk on people participating in other forms of gambling.

Here is a list of potential gambling behaviors that Shaffer and Martin believe might be risk factors to look out for in the development of problem gambling, with my additions in parentheses showing the connections to other drug addictions.

—**Betting Intensity**: how many bets per day. (With alcohol, how many drinks.)

—**Gambling Frequency**: number of gambling days (Number of drinking days.)

—**Gambling Trajectory**: tendency to increase the amount of wagered money. (Tolerance, in the case of drugs and alcohol.)

—**Gambling Variability**: deviation from consistent gambling pattern. (Inability to predict duration or outcome of drinking event.)

But if we list gambling under Addiction and Related Disorders, must we list all the possible variations on the theme—shopping and sex and all the rest, even though the picture is still fuzzy? No, the authors argue, we don't. Not right this minute. But gambling is ready to join the roster. Shaffer and Martin would like to see their syndrome model of addiction used to identify "core features of addiction and then illustrate these with substance-related and behavioral expressions of this diagnostic class. Conceptualizing addiction this way avoids the incorrect view that the object causes the addiction and shifts the diagnostic focus toward patient needs."

Saturday, June 25, 2011

http://addiction-dirkh.blogspot.com/2011/06/that-pesky-gambling-question.html

Shaffer HJ, & Martin R. Disordered gambling: etiology, trajectory, and clinical considerations. *Annual review of clinical psychology,* 7, 483-510. 2011. PMID: 21219194

Is Coumadin the Most Dangerous Drug in America?

Common drug most likely to land seniors in the hospital.

High-risk drugs for seniors aren't the ones you might think. Take warfarin, trade name Coumadin. Millions of seniors do. For people with certain kinds of heart trouble, or who have had a stroke, Coumadin works against the blood's tendency to clot, and saves lives. In cases of accidental overdose, however, it causes uncontrolled bleeding, and is the likeliest drug to put people over 65 in the emergency room. To further complicate matters, Warfarin interacts with a number of common medications, such as antibiotics, in ways that alter the blood's clotting ability.

A team of researchers from the Centers for Disease Control and Prevention (CDC) and Emory University studied almost 100,000 emergency hospitalizations due to adverse drug events between 2007 and 2009. **The results, published in the *New England Journal of Medicine*, showed that nearly two-thirds of such hospitalizations were due to hemorrhages caused by unintentional overdoses, and that warfarin was the leading culprit, accounting for about one third of the admissions and costing "hundreds of millions of dollars annually."** Prescription painkillers and sedatives, generally considered to be a major hazard for seniors, account for a mere fraction of hospital admissions—about 1.2%.

Accidental overdoses of insulin products came in second, followed closely by anti-coagulant drugs like Plavix and aspirin. The study makes clear that the main danger for seniors is hemorrhages and other forms of uncontrolled bleeding. **In addition, insulin overdose can cause fainting and seizures, and it is not uncommon for those over 65 to be taking drugs for both diabetes and heart disease at the same time.**

Half of those hospitalized for drug emergencies were over the age of 80, according to the study, which says that drug-related hospitalizations can only grow as the population ages. 40% of Americans over the age of 65 take five to nine medications, the study revealed.

Clearly, doctors can cut down on admissions and save money by more closely monitoring medications in older patients. But the sad fact is that physicians don't do a very good job of keeping track of all the medications older patients may be taking. Michael R. Cohen of the Institute for Safe Medication Practices told the *Wall Street Journal* that pharmacists needed to step into the information gap: "When you get a prescription filled, you're handed a patient education sheet that's a printout from the computer," he said. "It's very difficult to read, so it generally ends up in the trash."

Friday, December 2, 2011

http://addiction-dirkh.blogspot.com/2011/12/is-coumadin-most-dangerous-drug-in.html

Daniel S. Budnitz, M.D., M.P.H., Maribeth C. Lovegrove, M.P.H., Nadine Shehab, Pharm.D., M.P.H., and Chesley L. Richards, M.D., M.P.H Emergency Hospitalizations for Adverse Drug Events in Older Americans. New England Journal of Medicine. 2011; 365:2002-2012. 2011. DOI: 10.1056/NEJMsa1103053

Common Field Test for Marijuana is Unreliable, Critics Say

A 75-year old pot assay is due for an update.

We've all seen it on cop shows: The little plastic bag, the officer breaking the seal on a small pipette and inserting a bit of marijuana, then a firm shake, and voila, the liquid in the test satchel turns purple: Guilty.

Here's an interesting twist they don't tell you about: **The so-called Duquenois-Levine test—the dominant method for field-testing marijuana since 1930—is considered by many to be wildly inaccurate, and frequently doesn't hold up in court.** One U.S. Superior Court judge referred to the test as "pseudo-scientific."

The test itself works fine. The problem is that, in addition to identifying marijuana or hashish, the Duquenois-Levine, or D-L, frequently reads positive for tea, nutmeg, sage, and dozens of other chemicals—including resorcinols, a family of over-the-counter medicines, which, according to John Kelly at *AlterNet,* includes Sucrets throat lozenges. **This does matter, because in New York, Washington, D.C., and elsewhere, inner-city minority kids are getting busted for pot in record numbers.** Lacking a reliable test protocol, marijuana is whatever the officer says it is. In a classic case that continues to bedevil the testing industry, a middle-aged woman was busted for marijuana while

55

bird watching. A "leafy substance" turned purple on the Duquenois-Levine (D-L) test, and the woman was arrested. The material turned out to be sage, sweetgrass, and lavender, and the woman was engaging in a Native American purifying ritual using a smudge, a concept with which the arresting officers were unfamiliar.

So, when push comes to shove, a positive D-L rarely establishes the presence of marijuana beyond a reasonable doubt, without further confirmatory testing. For at least 20 years now, a visual inspection and a NarcoPouch, as the D-L field test is called, were enough to bring on the felony charges. State courts have squabbled over the matter, but state legislatures have been reluctant to intervene, in large part because sending samples to a lab for confirmatory testing is prohibitively expensive, particularly when the busts are small. The D-L test saves money.

According to the official drug policy of the United Nations, a positive marijuana ID requires gas chromatography/mass spectrometry analysis. And even this far more sophisticated test has angered courts in Washington and Colorado, the *UK Guardian* reports, "because the DEA doesn't have standard lab protocols to govern its use." In part, the judges are furious because plea-bargaining depends upon valid drug possession evidence. So, the officers themselves, when it comes to testifying in court, become de facto expert witnesses, able to identify illegal drugs on sight. Ah, those were the days. But now, cannabis-based products come in a bewildering variety of sizes, shapes, colors, smells, and chemical compositions.

But c'mon, if it looks like bud and it smells like bud... except that the research shows there are 120 terpenoid-type compounds involved in the odor of marijuana. No two varieties smell exactly alike. There *is* no characteristic marijuana smell—there are hundreds of characteristic marijuana smells. Nonetheless, in 2009 the National Academy of Sciences called the testing of controlled substances "a mature forensic science discipline," according to *AlterNet*.

In a 2008 article for the *Texas Tech Law Review*, Frederic Whitehurst, Executive Director for the Forensic Justice Project and formerly with the FBI, concluded: **"We are arresting vast numbers of citizens for possession of a substance that we cannot identify by utilizing the forensic protocol that is presently in use in most crime labs in the United States."** In another section of the article, Whitehurst asks: "Why is this protocol still being utilized to decide whether human beings should be confined to cages and at times, to death chambers?" And as Stewart J. Lawrence and John Kelly write in the *Guardian*, "using manifestly flawed drug identification tests to charge defendants, or pressure them to plead guilty, is hard to square with a defendant's right to due process."

Wednesday, August 10, 2011

http://addiction-dirkh.blogspot.com/2011/08/common-field-test-for-marijuana-is.html

For Smokers, Nowhere to Run and Nowhere to Hide

(With love and apologies to Martha and the Vandellas.)

That wonderful song goes on to declare:

> *'Cause I know*
> *You're no good for me*
> *But you've become*
> *A part of me.*

The song is not about cigarette addiction, but it could be. Full Disclosure: I smoked cigarettes myself for almost 25 years. And then, after several failed attempts, I quit. I out myself on this subject because a paper from the May 25 issue of the *New England Journal of Medicine* (NEJM) decries what the authors call the "denormalization" of smoking—and I find myself agreeing with them, smokeless though I may be. I recently visited New York, coincidentally on the day that smoking outdoors in New York City became illegal. Okay, that's not quite fair to say—it became illegal to smoke in Central Park, or at Brighton Beach, or along the newly pedestrian mallways of Times Square. There is no smoking along the High Line. **There is no smoking at any park, beach, or pedestrian mall. As both the tobacco industry and anti-smoking activists well know, this was an iconic victory that has the potential to change smoking laws in virtually every other American city.**

It's a fascinating progression, starting in the 70s when the Civil Aeronautics Board decreed non-smoking sections on domestic airline flights, to the recent New York City Council Decision to ban smoking *en plein air*, so to speak. Thomas Farley, New York City Health Commissioner, summed it up as follows in a public hearing: "I think in the future, we will look back on this time and say 'How could we have ever tolerated smoking in a park?'"

I'm not so sure on that, myself. James Colgrove, Ronald Bayer, and Kathleen Bachynski of the Mailman School of Public Health at Columbia University wrote the paper, entitled "Nowhere Left to Hide? The Banishment of Smoking from Public Spaces," in the NEJM. The authors note that more than 500 towns and cities in 43 different states have already enacted laws banning smoking "in outdoor recreation areas." **At first, as the authors summarize the history, it all seems like a sensible compromise, built on common courtesy. First airplanes and buses, then restaurants and bars, began setting aside seats for non-smokers.** By the early 90s, the first data on secondhand smoke was rolling in. Schools, convention centers, and finally even private workplaces either banned smoking or created smoke-free areas. But even then, the primary motivator, according to the researchers, was that secondhand smoke was "unpleasant and annoying," not deadly. Smokers weren't being asked to refrain from public smoking for the good of their own health, but as a courtesy to others.

The solid scientific evidence kept accumulating, however—even though tobacco cigarettes were, and still are, completely legal products for adult Americans to purchase and consume if they so choose. Now the arguments shifted to the innocent bystanders, those within the six-foot ring, the immediate smoke zone surrounding a smoker, and the elevated risk of lung cancer, heart disease, and asthma that smokers were subjecting them to. **In 1993, the Environmental Protection Agency (EPA) classified**

secondhand smoke as a Class A carcinogen, and more school, stadiums and offices proscribed smoking.

So far so good, really, from a public health standpoint. But now comes the bend in the road. Suddenly, parks and beaches were being added to the no-smoking roster. "As the zones of prohibition are extended from indoor to outdoor spaces, however, the evidence of physical harm to bystanders grows more tenuous." **In 2008, the authors report, "The editor of the journal** *Tobacco Control* **dismissed as 'flimsy' the evidence that secondhand smoke poses a threat to the health of nonsmokers in most outdoor settings."**

This confusion was much in evidence at public hearings last fall on the proposed outdoor smoking bans. While Health commissioner Farley argued that 57% of New Yorkers showed nicotine by-products in their blood, he also argued that exposing young children to adults in the carnal act of smoking was detrimental to the public health and welfare. "Families," he said, "should be able to bring their children to parks and beaches knowing that they won't see others smoking." This is really quite an astonishing assertion, given the range of bad habits youngsters are exposed to as they go about a normal day in the adult world. The authors are particularly concerned about this push to stigmatize smokers. "Given the addictive nature of nicotine and the difficultly of quitting smoking, strategies of denormalization raise both pragmatic and ethical concerns." Furthermore:

The decline in U.S. smoking rates since the 1960s has coincided with the development of a sharp gradient along the lines of socioeconomic status. Whereas about one fifth of all Americans are smokers, about one third of those with incomes below the federal poverty level smoke. These data are especially pertinent to the question of bans in parks. Since smokers are more likely to be poor and therefore dependent on free public spaces for enjoyment and recreation, refusing to allow them to smoke in those places poses potential problems of fairness.

The anti-tobacco movement, frustrated by the slow pace of gains over several years of active efforts, with rates of smoking remaining essentially unchanged, has to face the fact that an outright ban on cigarettes is a ticket to black market, crime syndicate hell. But a *de facto* ban is something altogether different, and "steadily winnowing the spaces in which smoking is legally allowed may be leading to a kind of de facto prohibition." More and more employers prohibit smoking in doorways, within ten feet of doorways, anywhere on university campuses, and so on. **No one has voted to make cigarette smoking illegal. But the public space in which this legal activity can be pursued is disappearing**. And here is where the tough questions start: "In the absence of direct health risks to others, bans on smoking in parks and beaches raise questions about the acceptable limits for government to impose on conduct," the authors conclude. Not to mention issues of personal autonomy, individual choice, and the stigma attached to addictive behavior. Perhaps the ACLU will soon take an interest in the civil rights of outdoor smokers, where the only health being hazarded is the smokers' own.

Friday, June 3, 2011

http://addiction-dirkh.blogspot.com/2011/06/for-smokers-nowhere-to-run-and-nowhere.html

Colgrove J, Bayer R, & Bachynski KE. Nowhere Left to Hide? The Banishment of Smoking from Public Spaces. *The New England Journal of Medicine*. (2011). PMID: 21612464

Impulsivity and Addiction

The perils of a hypersensitive dopamine system.

The brooding, antisocial loner, the one with impulse control problems, a penchant for risk-taking, and a cigarette dangling from his lip, is a recognizable archetype in popular culture. From Marlon Brando to Bruce Lee, these flawed heroes are perhaps the ones with restless brain chemicals; the ones who never felt good and never knew why ("What are you rebelling against?" "What've you got?").

A recent study at Vanderbilt University, published in *Nature Neuroscience*, used PET scans and fMRI imaging to suggest that impulsivity and other "antisocial" traits "predicted nucleus accumbens dopamine release and reward anticipation-related activity in response to pharmacological and monetary reinforcers, respectively."

In other words, the Vanderbilt researchers maintained that so-called "psychopathic traits" like impulsivity and risk taking are linked to addiction and gambling by means of an overly active dopamine system. PET scans of dopamine responses to a low dose of amphetamine showed that "individuals who scored high on a personality assessment that teases out traits like egocentricity, manipulating others, and risk taking had a hypersensitive dopamine response system," according to a press release from the National Institute on Drug Abuse (NIDA), which funded the study.

Putting a different spin on the matter, NIDA director Nora Volkow said: "By linking traits that suggest impulsivity and the potential for antisocial behavior to an overreactive dopamine system, this study helps explain why aggression may be as rewarding for some people as drugs are for others."

Lead author Joshua Buckholtz of Vanderbilt said that the amount of dopamine released was up to four times higher in people with high levels of these traits, compared to those who scored lower on the personality profile. Buckholtz suggested that a pattern of exaggerated dopamine responses "could develop into psychopathic personality disorder."

Dr. Robert Cloninger, a prominent addiction researcher, has asserted in the past that children who show a high propensity for risk-taking, along with impulsivity, or "novelty-seeking," are more likely to develop alcoholism and other addictions later in life.

And, in interviews with the late psychologist Henri Begleiter for my book on addiction science, Begleiter insisted that addicts were stuck with a package of symptoms he called behavioral dysregulation. "Disinhibition, impulsivity, trouble fitting into society— you have certain behavioral disorders in kids who later develop into alcoholics and drug addicts," he said. **The behavior itself doesn't cause the addiction. The dysregulated behavior is a symptom of the addiction."**

"When you talk to these people, as I have," Begleiter said, "you see that the one thing they pretty much all report is that, under the influence of the drug, they feel much more normal. It normalizes their central nervous systems. Initially, what they have is a need to experience a normal life."

So, it wasn't ducktails, pool halls, tattoos, casual sex, or lack of parental involvement that caused addiction to alcohol and cigarettes and pot, and maybe cocaine and speed and heroin. It wasn't just the "bad kids." **Irrational anger, impulsive decisions, certain compulsive behaviors like gambling—these behaviors**

were symptoms of the same group of related disorders that included drug and alcohol addiction, and which involved specific chemicals and areas of the brain related to reward, motivation, and memory.

The trait of impulsivity is a possible marker for addiction that may help explain why it is usually impossible to persuade addicts to give up their drugs by sheer force of logic—by arguing that the drugs will eventually ruin their health or kill them. "They tell me it'll kill me," sang Dave Van Ronk, "but they don't say when."

Consider the always-instructive case of cigarette smoking. In 1964, the Surgeon General's Report on Smoking and Health laid out the case for the long-term ill effects of nicotine quite effectively—and millions of people quit smoking. A stubborn minority did not, and many of them still have not. Are they simply being hedonistic and irresponsible? Or are the long-term negative consequences, so dramatically clear to others, simply not capable of influencing their thinking to the same degree? Biochemical abnormalities similar to those predisposing certain people to addiction may also prevent them from comprehending the long-term results of their behavior.

Tuesday, April 6, 2010

http://addiction-dirkh.blogspot.com/2010/04/impulsivity-and-addiction.html

Buckholtz, J., Treadway, M., Cowan, R., Woodward, N., Benning, S., Li, R., Ansari, M., Baldwin, R., Schwartzman, A., Shelby, E., Smith, C., Cole, D., Kessler, R., & Zald, D. Mesolimbic dopamine reward system hypersensitivity in individuals with psychopathic traits Nature Neuroscience, 13 (4), 419-421 (2010). DOI: 10.1038/nn.2510

Anandamide Hits the "Hedonic Hot Spot"

Marijuana and the munchies.

It's no secret that marijuana very reliably increases appetite. Recently, research published in *Nature* has teased out an apparent mechanism by which internal cannabinoids are involved with gut microbiota. This affects inflammation, the metabolism of adipose tissue, and other factors implicated in obesity.

In addition, research published in the Proceedings of the National Academy of Sciences, and blogged about by Neuroskeptic, showed that CB1 cannabinoid receptors on the tongue selectively boost our pleasurable responses to sweet-tasting food. Conversely, drugs that block cannabinoid receptors have been actively pursued as appetite suppressants. **One such drug, trade name rimonabant, was disallowed by the FDA on the grounds that it worked so well in the guise of anandamide's opposite number that it frequently caused debilitating depression in users.** But it did appear to reduce appetites.

Neuroskeptic suggests that a CB1 antagonist that only affects specific sites, like taste buds, might be able to lessen the sweet-tooth effect with fewer complications. "Who knows," he writes, "in a few years you might even be able to buy CB1 antagonist chewing gum to help you stick to your diet."

We know that cannabinoids make rats and humans eat more. But how, exactly, does that happen? One reasonable hypothesis is that anandamide, other endocannabinoids, and cannabinoid drugs—anything that tickles the CB1 receptors–must increase sensations of palatability, if eaters are to eat more. A group of University of Michigan researchers chose to investigate the theory that "endogenous cannabinoid neurotransmission in limbic structures such as nucleus accumbens mediates the hedonic impact of natural rewards like sweetness." **They went looking for the precise brain location—the "hedonic hotspot for sensory pleasure"—where endocannabinoids do their work.**

Writing in *Neuropsychopharmacology* in 2007, the investigators sought to discover "if anandamide microinjection into medial nucleus accumbens shell enhances these affective reactions to sweet and bitter tastes in rats." And it did. Anandamide "doubled the number of positive 'liking' reactions elicited by intraoral sucrose, without altering negative 'disliking' reactions to bitter quinine." Anandamide reliably increased the number of "positive hedonic reactions" the rats showed to sucrose, and never caused any aversive reactions, or increases in water drinking or other behaviors. In addition, the process worked in reverse: "Food-related manipulations, such as deprivation and satiety, or access to a palatable diet produce changes in CB1 receptor density," leading to higher levels of endogenous anandamide.

One location in particular, when dosed with endocannabinoids, increased "liking" responses in the rats threefold. **A tiny spot, 1.6 millimeters cubed, but the hottest spot of all: the dorsal half of the medial shell of the nucleus accumbens. At that site, cannabinoid receptors and opioid receptors appear to coexist and interact.** If this form of colocalization occurs regularly in rats and humans, it would constitute strong support for the idea that "endocannabinoid and opioid neurochemical signals in the nucleus accumbens might interact to enhance 'liking' reactions to the sensory pleasure of sucrose."

As the authors sum it up, "magnifying the pleasurable impact of food reward" appears to be the baseline effect of endocannabinoids on "appetite or incentive motivation." Because all of this takes place along the brain's primary reward pathways in the limbic system, the authors conclude that it would be of interest to know "whether other types of sensory pleasure besides sweetness can be enhanced by the endocannabinoid hedonic hotspot described here."

Tuesday, October 26, 2010

http://addiction-dirkh.blogspot.com/2010/10/
anandamide-hits-hedonic-hot-spot.html

Mahler, S., Smith, K., & Berridge, K. Endocannabinoid Hedonic Hotspot for Sensory Pleasure: Anandamide in Nucleus Accumbens Shell Enhances 'Liking' of a Sweet Reward *Neuropsychopharmacology*, *32* (11), 2267-2278. 2007. DOI: 10.1038/sj.npp.1301376

The Perils of Fair-Weather Cocaine

The higher the temp, the higher the death rate.

Cocaine users might want to take note of further evidence of a connection between high ambient air temperatures and accidental overdoses.

A study published recently in the journal *Addiction* used mortality data from the Office of the Chief Medical Examiner in New York City from 1990 to 2006 to determine the frequency of cocaine-related overdoses (itself an enterprise fraught with uncertainty and argument over listed causes of death). The researchers cross-referenced the mortality data with temperature records from the National Oceanic and Atmospheric Association (NOAA).

As reported in *Addiction Journal*, "accidental overdose deaths that were wholly or partly attributable to cocaine use rose significantly as the weekly ambient temperature passed 24 degrees Celsius [75 degrees F]."

Previous research, the authors write, had indicated that significantly higher temperatures—in the high 80s F—were required before cocaine mortality rates showed an increase. **The researchers said they did not detect a corresponding rise in other types of drug overdoses during days over 75 degrees.**

What is the mechanism connecting temperature to cocaine overdose? Cocaine intoxication raises core body temperature. **Overheated cocaine users risk overdosing on smaller doses of the drug**

because their bodies are already under the strain of mild hyperthermia, or increased body temperature.

Specifically, the researchers from the University of Michigan and elsewhere found that above 75 degrees, there were 0.25 more drug overdoses per 1,000,000 residents per week for every two-degree rise in temperature, according to *Addiction Journal*. **Applied to New York City, these numbers suggest and additional two cocaine deaths per week for every two degrees increase in average temperature over 75.**

Lead author Dr. Amy Bohnert of the University of Michigan Medical School said in a press release that cocaine users are already "at a high risk of negative health outcomes and need public health attention, particularly when the weather is warm." During the study period, New York City had average weekly temperatures in the >24 C range roughly seven weeks per year.

The idea is quite plausible, given that ambient air temperature can affect many other metabolic processes. Earlier investigations led to the discovery of a fairly well established diurnal AND seasonal variation for measurements of blood pressure. Researchers at Emory University data-mined 2 million electronic records of participating patients and discovered that the odds of having high blood pressure were lowest during the morning, and generally increased throughout the day. Seasonally, high blood pressure occurred more often in winter, and was at its lowest in the summer.

Sunday, March 7, 2010

http://addiction-dirkh.blogspot.com/2010/03/perils-of-fair-weather-cocaine.html

Bohnert, A., Prescott, M., Vlahov, D., Tardiff, K., & Galea, S. Ambient temperature and risk of death from accidental drug overdose in New York City, 1990-2006 *Addiction*. 2010. DOI: 10.1111/j.1360-0443.2009.02887.x

Does Brain Research Worsen the Addiction Stigma?

"Once an addict, always an addict."

When it comes to the neurobiology of addiction, the research community has made great strides in a few hectic years. However, as addiction counselor William White wrote in 2007, are we lacking a comparable neurobiology of addiction *recovery*?

White, a senior research consultant at Chestnut Health Systems/Lighthouse Institute, warns that in the past, **campaigns seeking to reduce the stigma of mental illness by educating the public about "brain disease" have often inadvertently backfired, and invoked, instead, "harsher behavior toward the mentally ill."**

White states the matter starkly: "The vivid brain images of the addicted person may make that person's behavior more understandable, but they do not make the person whose brain is being scanned more desirable as a friend, lover, spouse, neighbor, or employee."

Furthermore, writes White, emphasizing the "chronic" part of a chronic brain disease can mislead the public into believing, "once an addict, always an addict."

What can be done to balance out the downside of public perceptions related to the brain disease of addiction? White suggests that what is missing is what he refers to as the neurobiology of addiction recovery. When we convey to people that addiction is a brain disease that "alters emotional affect, compromises judgment, impairs memory, inhibits one's capacity for new learning, and erodes behavioral impulse control," we are not always helping to reduce the stigma of the disorder.

This state of affairs will continue, says White "unless there are two companion communications: 1) With abstinence and proper care, addiction-induced brain impairments rapidly reverse themselves, and 2) millions of individuals have achieved complete long-term recovery from addiction and have gone on to experience healthy, meaningful, and productive lives."

White points out the lack of a specific research agenda in the field of addiction science that focuses on the "prevalence, pathways, styles and stages of LONG-TERM recovery." Specifically, a comprehensive research agenda would need to include answers to question such as:

—**"To what degree does neurobiology influence who recovers from addiction and who does not achieve such recovery?"**

—**"What is the time period over which such pathologies are reversed in recovery—days, months, years?"**

—**"What role can pharmacological adjuncts, social support and other services play in extending and speeding this process of brain recovery?"**

—**"Are there critical differences in the extent and timing of neurobiological recovery related to age of onset of use... age of onset of recovery, gender, genetic load for addiction, developmental trauma", and other factors?**

Thursday, November 26, 2009

http://addiction-dirkh.blogspot.com/2009/11/does-brain-research-worsen-addiction_26.html

White's paper, "In Search of the Neurobiology of Addiction Recovery: A Brief Commentary on Science and Stigma." http://www.facesandvoicesofrecovery.org/resources/publications_white.php

When Smokers Move

Is your new house a thirdhand smoke reservoir?

In the first published examination of thirdhand smoke pollution and exposure, researchers at San Diego State University discovered that non-smokers who move into homes purchased from smokers encounter significantly elevated nicotine levels in the air and dust of their new homes two months or more after moving in.

100 smoking households and 50 non-smoking households participated in the study, which was published in *Tobacco Control*. The researchers tested for surface nicotine levels in living rooms and bedrooms, took finger nicotine concentrations, collected dust and air samples, and measured urine concentrations of the nicotine breakdown product cotinine.

So, what faces non-smoking new homeowners when they take up residence in a smoker's former home? "Air nicotine concentrations were 35-98 times higher than those found in non-smoker homes," the investigators write. **"Dust and surfaces showed nicotine levels approximately 12-21 and 30-150 times higher, respectively, than the reference levels in non-smoker homes."**

The homes had been vacated a median of 62 days, and tests on the new residents were conducted a median of 34 days after the move. "Nicotine levels found on the index fingers of non-smokers residing in former smoker homes were 7-8 times higher" than those residing in non-smoking homes. What makes this even more noteworthy is that most of the smokers' homes "underwent cleaning and many were repainted and had carpets replaced before new occupants moved in." **In addition, "smoker homes remained vacant for on average an extra month," all of which suggests that smoking has a host of economic side effects we are only beginning to pin down.**

"In summary," say the researchers, "these findings demonstrate that smokers leave behind a legacy of thirdhand smoke (THS) in the dust and on the surfaces of their homes that persists over weeks and months." But do these numbers rise to the level of a legitimate health and safety concern? After all, an exposure of 150 times more cigarette smoke than the background nicotine pollution level of essentially zero doesn't necessarily mean a hazardous layer of left-over smoke.

Unless, possibly, you happen to be a small child who likes to crawl around on everything you can reach, wearing only your diapers, while licking absolutely everything you come across and simultaneously "ingesting non-food items," as the researchers put it. In that case, your exposure to the nicotine, phenol, cresols, naphthalene, formaldehyde, and tobacco-specific nitrosamines (all combining in unknown ways with other pollutants and oxidants in the home environment), and the potential effect of that exposure on your immature immune system, might be high enough to raise the concern level of your parents.

Sunday, April 3, 2011

http://addiction-dirkh.blogspot.com/2011/04/when-smokers-move.html

Matt, G., Quintana, P., Zakarian, J., Fortmann, A., Chatfield, D., Hoh, E., Uribe, A., & Hovell, M. When smokers move out and non-smokers move in: residential thirdhand smoke pollution and exposure *Tobacco Control, 20* (1). 2010. DOI: 10.1136/tc.2010.037382

Modafinil May Be Addictive

NIDA study casts doubt on safety of "brain booster" drug.

Despite the headlines, most new drugs are not addictive. Very few medications show the distinctive side effects associated with clinical drug addiction: tolerance, withdrawal, and continued use despite adverse consequences. Such drugs are relatively rare—so it was with interest and alarm that addiction specialists confronted a small pilot study, led by Dr. Nora Volkow of the National Institute on Drug Abuse (NIDA), which appeared to demonstrate that the sleep drug modafinil has addictive potential.

Modafinil, sold as Provigil, has found increasing off-prescription use for the treatment of ADHD and other psychiatric disorders. The drug is also being used as a so-called "cognitive enhancement" drug or "brain booster," particularly among college students and military field personnel. Modafinil had even shown early promise as a drug for the treatment of cocaine addiction.

In the March 18 issue of the *Journal of the American Medical Association* (JAMA), the researchers reported on levels of extracellular dopamine in the brains of 10 healthy men on either placebo or modafinil.

According to the researchers, "Modafinil acutely increased dopamine levels and blocked dopamine transporters in the human brain. Because drugs that increase dopamine have the potential for abuse, and considering the increasing use of modafinil for multiple purposes, these results suggest that risk for addiction in vulnerable persons merits heightened awareness."

Scientists were initially excited about a drug which showed stimulant properties but did not appear to have a direct effect on the dopamine pleasure systems of the brain—a finding that set it apart from drugs like amphetamine and cocaine. However, as reported online by Heidi Ledford of *Nature*, "Animal studies showed that rodents that lack dopamine receptors are unresponsive to the drug, and in 2006, researchers found that modafinil affects dopamine levels in the brains of rhesus macaques."

Dr. Volkow stressed that patients taking modafinil for recognized medical conditions such as narcolepsy should continue to do so, while doctors should monitor modafinil patients for signs of dependency.

Still, dopamine is not all there is to addiction. As reported in *Nature*, Bertha Madras of Harvard Medical School notes that some drugs that boost dopamine have other properties that make them aversive, and therefore not addictive. "The full spectrum of the pharmacology of the drug is what drives the abuse potential," she said.

Wednesday, March 18, 2009

http://addiction-dirkh.blogspot.com/2009/03/modafinil-may-be-addictive.html

Ledford, Heidi. Cognitive enhancement drug may also cause addiction. *Nature*. 17 March 2009. doi:10.1038/news.2009.170

Does Menthol Really Matter?

Nicotine experts say menthol makes addiction more likely but differ over what to do about it.

Back in the 1920s, Lloyd "Spud" Hughes of Mingo Junction, Ohio, was working as a restaurant cashier when, legend has it, he smoked some cigarettes that had been casually stored in a tin that contained menthol crystals. Menthol, a compound found in mint plants and also manufactured synthetically, is used medicinally, and as a food flavoring. Back in Spud's day, menthol was mostly derived by extracting crystals from the Japanese Mint plant. **What we know for certain is that the mentholated cigarettes tasted so good to Spud that he patented the mixture.** In 1925, the Spud Cigarette Corporation of Wheeling, West Virginia, was born, and Spud Cigarettes quickly became the 5th best selling cigarette brand in America.

Dr. Neal L. Benowitz, Professor of Medicine and Bioengineering & Therapeutic Sciences, and Chief of the Division of Clinical Pharmacology at the University of California in San Francisco, says that Spud Hughes had "accidentally identified an additive whose pharmacologic actions reduce the irritating properties of smoke generally and nicotine specifically." Menthol accomplishes this because it acts on receptors involved in the detection of physical stimuli like temperature and chemical irritation. **"Menthol contributes to perceptions of cigarettes' strength, harshness,**

or mildness, smoothness, coolness, taste, and aftertaste." That would seem to just about cover it. But no: In their article for the *New England Journal Of Medicine*—"The Threat of Menthol Cigarettes to U.S. Public Health"—Benowitz and Jonathan M. Samet also claim that "menthol has druglike characteristics that interact at the receptor level with the actions of nicotine."

And nicotine hardly needs much help establishing its grip over addiction-prone individuals. "It's not that it's so intensive," Dr. Benowitz told me some years ago, when I was researching my book, *The Chemical Carousel*, "it's just that it's so reliable. Nicotine arouses you in the morning; it relaxes you in the afternoon. It's a drug that you can dose many times per day for the purpose of modulating your mood, and it becomes highly conditioned, more than any other drug, because it's used every single day, multiple times per day."

Benowitz, along with Dr. Michael Siegel of the Boston University School of Public Health, recently sparked intense debate when they both championed electronic cigarettes as a safe alternative to smoking tobacco cigarettes, despite the FDA's earlier wish to keep e-cigarettes out of the country. And last month, an advisory report for the FDA by a group that included Benowitz and Samet concluded that mentholated cigarettes were no more harmful, and no more likely to cause disease, than regular cigarettes. A study in the *Journal of the National Cancer Institute* of 440 lung cancer patients and more than 2,000 matched patients without lung cancer showed no correlation at all between menthol and cancer. In fact, the researchers were surprised to discover that menthol smokers appear to have a lower risk of lung cancer than other smokers. Asked whether menthol cigarettes are more toxic than non-menthol cigarettes, the study's author William Blot of Vanderbilt University definitively responded: "The answer is, no, they are not."

However, the advisory report suggested that, while menthol cigarettes may not be more dangerous, they might be more *addictive* than regular cigarettes. In the May 4 *New England Journal of Medicine* article, Benowitz and Samet argue that because menthol cigarettes attract younger smokers by making tobacco easier to smoke, and because more of these smokers go on to become lifelong nicotine addicts due to this same cooling effect, "menthol cigarettes increase the likelihood of addiction and the degree of addiction in new smokers." Further adding to menthol's tendency to create lifelong smokers is the fact that "some consumers, particularly blacks, hold beliefs about implicit health benefits of menthol cigarettes that may interfere with their quitting."

This is a substantial indictment of menthol as a component of cigarettes, despite the belief among some experts that it is much ado about nothing. But if that's the case, Benowitz and Samet suggest, why has the tobacco industry fought so ferociously to exempt menthol from the list of banned flavorings over the years? **And why has the industry so consistently linked its marketing of menthol cigarettes to images of "freshness" and health?** The authors estimated that "by 2020 about 17,000 more premature deaths will have occurred and two million more people will have started smoking than would have been the case if menthol cigarettes were not available." **Two million additional cigarette smokers by the end of the decade does not sound especially trivial.** Nonetheless, the FDA advisory report that Benowitz helped to shape stopped short of recommending an outright ban on nicotine, saying only that removal of menthol would "benefit public health."

While not disputing the findings of the FDA Advisory Committee, Dr. Michael Siegel of Boston University expressed dismay that "despite these conclusions, the [committee] did not recommend a ban

on menthol cigarettes." There are almost 20 million menthol smokers in the U.S., Siegel argues. If even a fraction of them quite smoking due to a ban on menthol in cigarettes, "it would have a profound effect on public health." This is, Siegel insists, precisely why politicians managed to exempt menthol from bans on various flavor additives in the first place. The Black Congressional Caucus had "vigorously denounced the exclusion of menthol" at the time, while Lorillard, maker of Newports—the leading brand of menthol cigarettes—argued that banning menthol would result in the creation of a huge black market. Because of all this, Seigel charges, Benowitz and the committee simply "punted the issue back to the FDA." And if anyone harbored doubts about who benefited from this non-action, in Siegel's view, one need only look at the fact that Lorillard's stock enjoyed a nice run-up of about 8% after the public announcement of the FDA panel's recommendations.

Because of all this, Siegel does not believe the FDA will ever ban menthol cigarettes. In his view, the Obama administration doesn't need the grief of added health care complexities just now, and there is no movement in Congress to make additives an issue. **And since the FDA has chosen not to demand the banning of menthol, Siegel thinks the committee's findings will serve as a convenient smokescreen for Congress.** And for the makers of menthol cigarettes, it will be business as usual. A window of opportunity on the menthol issue is now closing, says Siegel, who confesses to difficulty understanding a policy that bans "every other type of cigarette flavoring—including chocolate, strawberry, banana, pineapple, cherry, and kiwi—yet exempts the one flavoring that is actually used extensively by tobacco companies to recruit and maintain smokers... Menthol is a major contributor to smoking initiation and continued addiction, and for this reason, it will continue to enjoy the protection of a federal government that seems afraid to alienate any corporation, whether it's part of Big Pharma, Big Insurance, or Big Tobacco."

Friday, May 13, 2011

http://addiction-dirkh.blogspot.com/2011/05/
does-menthol-really-matter.html

Siegel, Michael. A Lost Opportunity for Public Health — The FDA Advisory Committee Report on Menthol. *New England Journal of Medicine*. 364:2177-2179 June 9, 2011. DOI: 10.1056/ NEJMp1103403

Marijuana and Memory

Do certain strains make you more forgetful?

Cannabis snobs have been known to argue endlessly about the quality of the highs produced by their favorite varietals: Northern Lights, Hawaiian Haze, White Widow, etc. Among dedicated potheads, debates about the effects of specific cannabis strains are often overheated, and, ultimately, kind of boring. It's a bit like listening to a discussion of whether the wine in question evinces a woody aftertaste or is, instead, redolent of elderberries. For most people, the true essence of wine drinking is pretty straightforward: a drug buzz, produced by a 12 to 15 % concentration of ethyl alcohol derived from grapes, which can be had in a spectrum of varietal flavors.

However, there is no doubting that, unlike the case of wine, different strains of marijuana can have markedly different psychoactive effects. With weed, it's not just a matter of taste.

Over the past couple of years, the cannabis debate has taken a nasty turn, after British scientists published several controversial studies suggesting that high-THC "skunk" cannabis was responsible for increased mental problems among young people—including an increased risk of developing the symptoms of schizophrenia. British drug policy makers have continued to lead the charge on this, with mixed results.

Recently, a study published in the *British Journal Of Psychiatry* concluded that marijuana high in THC—including so-called "skunk" cannabis—caused markedly more memory impairment than varieties of marijuana containing less THC.

In an article at *Nature News*, Arran Frood spelled out the details of the study:

"Curran and her colleagues traveled to the homes of 134 volunteers, where the subjects got high on their own supply before completing a battery of psychological tests designed to measure anxiety, memory recall and other factors such as verbal fluency when both sober and stoned. The researchers then took a portion of the stash back to the laboratory to test how much THC and cannabidiol it contained.... Analysis showed that participants who had smoked cannabis low in cannabidiol were significantly worse at recalling text than they were when not intoxicated. Those who smoked cannabis high in cannabidiol showed no such impairment."

The two main ingredients in cannabis are THC and cannabidiol (CBD). CBD shows less affinity for the two main types of cannabis receptors, CB1 and CB2, meaning that it attaches to receptors more weakly, and activates them less robustly, than THC. **The euphoric effects of marijuana are generally attributed to THC content, not CBD content. In fact, there appears to be an inverse ratio at work.** According to a paper in *Neuropsychopharmacology*, "Delta-9-THC and CBD can have opposite effects on regional brain function, which may underlie their different symptomatic and behavioral effects, and CBD's ability to block the psychotogenic effects of delta-9-THC."

So, CBD specifically does *not* produce the usual marijuana high with accompanying euphoria and forgetfulness and munchies. What the researchers found was that pot smokers suffering memory impairment and those showing normal memory "did not differ in the THC content of the cannabis they smoked. Unlike the marked impairment in prose recall of individuals who smoked cannabis low in cannabidiol, participants smoking cannabis high in cannabidiol showed no memory impairment."

As far as memory goes, THC content didn't seem to matter. It was the percentage of CBD that controlled the degree of memory impairment, the authors concluded. "The antagonistic effects of cannabidiol at the CB1 receptor are probably responsible for its profile in smoked cannabis, attenuating the memory-impairing effects of THC. In terms of harm reduction, users should be made aware of the higher risk of memory impairment associated with smoking low-cannabidiol strains of cannabis like 'skunk' and encouraged to use strains containing higher levels of cannabidiol."

The idea that cannabidiol may protect against THC-induced memory loss is still quite speculative. Other research has suggested that a paucity of CB1 receptors may be protective against memory impairment. Marijuana growers select for high-THC strains, not high-CBD strains, and thus there is little data available about the CBD levels of most marijuana.

An earlier study in *Behavioural Pharmacology* by Aaron Ilan and others at the San Francisco Brain Research Institute did not find any connection between memory and CBD content. However, Ilan speculated in the *Nature News* article that the difference might have been due to methodology: In Britain, the subjects were studied using marijuana of their own choosing. In the U.S., National Institute of Health research policy has decreed that marijuana for official research must be supplied by the National Institute on Drug Abuse (NIDA). And if there is one thing many researchers seem to agree on, it is that NIDA weed "is notorious for being low in THC and poor quality."

But CBD still does something, and that something just might be pain relief. Lester Grinspoon, a long-time marijuana researcher at Harvard Medical School, thinks that if the study proves out, it could have an important impact on the medical use of marijuana. Also quoted in *Nature News*, Grinspoon said: "Cannabis with high cannabidiol levels will make a more appealing option for anti-pain, anti-anxiety and anti-spasm treatments, because they can be delivered without causing disconcerting euphoria."

Sunday, October 3, 2010

http://addiction-dirkh.blogspot.com/2010/10/marijuana-and-memory.html

Morgan, C., Schafer, G., Freeman, T., & Curran, H. Impact of cannabidiol on the acute memory and psychotomimetic effects of smoked cannabis: naturalistic study *The British Journal of Psychiatry, 197* (4), 285-290. 2010. DOI: 10.1192/bjp.bp.110.077503

Drug-Drug Interactions to Watch Out For

P450 enzymes and "poor metabolizers."

The finding, published in *Science*, is a bit arcane to the layperson. The big secret of how the P450 enzyme family metabolizes drugs turns out to be a critical phase change, where an oxygen molecule temporarily joins the mix, forming "Compound I," a process the scientists documented by cooling the enzymes at just the right rate.

So what? Well, for starters, "cytochrome P450 enzymes are responsible for the phase I metabolism of approximately 75% of known pharmaceuticals," write Jonathan Rittle and Michael T. Green at Pennsylvania State University's Department of Chemistry. And in fact, only six of the more than 50 enzymes in the P450 family account for 90% of drug metabolization in humans—the compound known as CYP2D6 being the most crucial.

In a Penn State press release, lead author Michael Green, an associate professor of chemistry, noted that human populations vary widely in the version of genes they carry for P450 enzymes. According to Green, "adverse drug-drug interactions are a well-known problem.... Now that we can see those state changes on a molecular level, a deeper investigation is possible."

The wide variation in enzymatic reactions, says Green, causes very real consequences. People with two copies of variant alleles are poor metabolizers, people with two copies of the standard genetic variety are normal metabolizers, whereas people with one of each are "reduced" metabolizers. (People who inherit multiple copies of the alleles become "ultrarapid" metabolizers.)

"With a drug such as caffeine, for example, one population of people might be fast metabolizers, while another might metabolize the drug more slowly," Green said. "Because the risk of caffeine-induced heart attack may be higher in slow metabolizers, the ability to actually take a snapshot of the phase changes of the P450 enzymes could help us to understand better how certain chemicals can affect people in vastly different ways."

There are dozens of specific cases like the caffeine example. Moreover, the genetic situation is complicated by other factors. Writing in *American Family Physician,* Tom Lynch and Amy Price explain that cytochrome P450 enzymes "can be inhibited or induced by drugs, resulting in clinically significant drug-drug interactions that can cause unanticipated adverse reactions or therapeutic failures. **Interactions with warfarin, antidepressants, antiepileptic drugs, and statins often involve the cytochrome P450 enzymes.**"Testing for these interactions is expensive, and "it has not been determined if routine use of these tests will improve outcomes."

Not a pretty picture. And to further complicate matters, some drugs can induce or inhibit CYP450 enzymes differentially, depending upon the dosage. **"For instance," write Lynch and Price, "sertraline (Zoloft) is considered a mild inhibitor of CYP2D6 at a dose of 50 mg, but if the dose is increased to 200 mg, it becomes a potent inhibitor.** Inhibitory effects usually occur immediately." Also, drugs can be metabolized by, and at the same time serve to inhibit, the enzyme in question, as in the case of erythromycin.

So it is buyer beware, and listen to your body's feedback when embarking on a course of new drugs. **Recommended dosages are just that: recommendations.** If you feel that the drug in question is doing too much or too little, ask your prescribing doctor about drug-drug interactions and about fast and slow drug metabolizers. Of course, they should be telling YOU about that, but.

<u>**Some known enzymatic drug interactions to bear in mind:**</u>

Drugs that potentially inhibit P450 enzymes—Tagamet, Cipro, Luvox, Prozac, Flagyl, Benadryl, Paxil, Lamisil, and grapefruit juice.

Drugs that potentially increase the activity of P450 enzymes—Tegretol, phenobarbital, tobacco, Dilantin, rifampin, St. John's wort.

———

<u>**Adverse drug-drug interactions involving P450 enzymes:**</u>

Amiodarone (Cordarone) combined with Warfarin (Coumadin): possible bleeding due to increased warfarin activity.

Tegretol, phenobarbital, and Dilantin combined with contraceptives containing ethinyl estradiol: possible unplanned pregnancies due to reduced contraceptive activity.

Clarithromycin, erythromycin, and telithromycin combined with Zocor: possible muscle disorders due to increased Zocor levels.

Prozac combined with Risperidone (Risperdal): increased risk of adverse effects from the antipsychotic drug risperidone.

Grapefruit juice combined with Buspirone (Buspar): Dizziness and other effects of "serotonin syndrome" due to increased buspirone activity.

Monday, November 22, 2010

http://addiction-dirkh.blogspot.com/2010/11/drug-drug-interactions-to-watch-out-for.html

Rittle, J., & Green, M. Cytochrome P450 Compound I: Capture, Characterization, and C-H Bond Activation Kinetics *Science, 330* (6006), 933-937. 2010. DOI: 10.1126/science.1193478

Why are Treatment Centers Afraid of Anti-Craving Medications?

Using What Works.

Why do so many drug treatment centers continue to shun science by ignoring medications that ease the burden of withdrawal for many addicts? That's the question posed in an article by Alison Knopf in the May-June 2011 issue of *Addiction Professional*, titled "The Medication Holdouts."

"Nowhere else in medicine," Knopf writes, "are the people who treat a condition so suspicious of the very medications designed to help the condition in which they specialize."

Acamprosate, a drug used to treat alcoholism, is a good case in point. A dozen European studies examining thousands of alcohol test subjects found that the drug increased the number of days that most subjects were able to remain abstinent. But when a German drug maker decided to market the drug in the U.S., fierce advocates for drug-free addiction therapy came out in force, even though the drug was ultimately approved for use.

Disulfiram, naltrexone, acamprosate, methadone, buprenorphine—the evidence for all of them is solid. Knopf cites the case of buprenorphine:

"'There are scores of peer-reviewed journal articles that evaluate the success of buprenorphine," says Nicholas Reuter, MPH, senior public health adviser in the Division of Pharmacologic Therapies at the federal Center for Substance Abuse Treatment (CSAT). "It's well established that the data and the evidence are there." Not treating patients with a medication consigns most of them to relapse, adds Reuter. While some opioid-addicted patients, as many as 20 percent, do respond to abstinence-based therapy, 'That still leaves us with the 80 percent who don't,' he says.

Dr. Charles O'Brien, one the nation's most respected addiction professionals and a Professor of Psychiatry at the University of Pennsylvania, is incensed that anti-craving medications are not more widely used. **"It's unethical not to use medications," he says.** "This is a subject that I feel very strongly about." O'Brien told *Addiction Professional* he no longer cares who he offends on the subject. "If you're discouraging people from taking medications, you are behaving in an unethical way; you are depriving your patients of a way to turn themselves around. Just because you don't like it doesn't mean you have to keep your patients away from it."

And at the Association for Addiction Professionals, "the prevailing philosophy is pro-medication," Knopf writes. Misti Storie, education and training consultant for the group, told Knopf that the "disconnect" at treatment centers is due to a "lack of education about the connection between biology and addiction." Counselors working in centers that do not allow anti-craving medications are in a tough spot, Storie acknowledged.

It is continually astonishing that treatment centers–where the primary goal is supposed to be the prevention of relapse, even though the success rate remains abysmal–would spurn medications that often help to accomplish precisely that goal. **Relapse rates hover around 80%, by an amalgam of estimates, so it's not**

like rehabs are wildly successful at what they do. What's really behind the resistance?

What stands between many addicts and the new forms of treatment is "pharmacological Calvinism." I would love to claim this term as my own, but it was coined by Cornell University researcher Gerald Klerman. **Pharmacological Calvinism may be defined as the belief that treating any psychological symptoms with a pill is tantamount to ethical surrender, or, at the very least, a serious failure of will.** As Peter Kramer quoted Klerman in *Listening to Prozac*: If a drug makes you feel better, then by definition "somehow it is morally wrong and the user is likely to suffer retribution with either dependence, liver damage, or chromosomal change, or some other form of medical-theological damnation."

Sunday, June 12, 2011

http://addiction-dirkh.blogspot.com/2011/06/why-are-treatment-centers-afraid-of.html

Chasing the Genes for Cocaine Addiction

Brain protein MeCP2 in the spotlight.

Dr. Edward Sellers, former director of the psychopharmacological research program at the University of Toronto's Addiction Research Foundation, once said to me: "Every cell, every hormone, every membrane in the body has got genetic underpinnings, and while many of the genetic underpinnings are similar in people, in fact there are also huge differences. So on one level, the fact that there is a genetic component to addiction is not very surprising. What is surprising is that you could ever have it show up in a dominant enough way to be something that might be useful in anticipating risk."

If there existed a set of genes that predisposed people to alcoholism, and possibly other addictions, then these genes had to control the expression of something specific. That's what genes did. However, back in the 1990s, addiction researchers could not even agree on the matter of where they should be looking for such physical evidence of genetic difference. In the brain? Among the digestive enzymes? Blood platelets? A gene, or a set of genes, coding for… what? What was it they were supposed to be looking for?

What set of genes coded for addiction?

Something about modern genetic research breeds a strong jolt of excitement. There is the promise of sudden discoveries, headlines, and great leaps forward toward cures for stubborn diseases.

Even the most sober scientists seem to get enthused about gene hunting. **The idea of curing a disease by locating a defective gene and repairing it is one of the brightest and fondest hopes in medicine.** At least 3,000 medical disorders, including diabetes, cystic fibrosis, and some forms of Alzheimer's are inherited diseases caused by defective genes passed on from generation to generation. But the premature announcements and retractions involving genes for everything from drinking to shyness has brought a hard-won maturity to the field.

These days, the hunt for evidence of genes influencing addiction is drilling very deeply into the molecular underpinnings of neural activity, in a wide-ranging effort to sort out the variety of gene interactions involved in the genetic propensity for alcoholism and other addictions.

Work done at the Scripps Research Institute in Florida, funded by the National Institute on Drug Abuse (NIDA) and published in *Nature Neuroscience*, recently shone a spotlight on a gene responsible for making a particular protein—MeCP2—needed for normal development of nerve cells in the brain. This gene for methyl CpG binding protein 2 is best known as the gene responsible for a rare genetic brain disorder called Rett syndrome.

Researchers at Scripps discovered that cocaine increased levels of this regulatory protein in the brains of rats. So did fluoxetine , better known as Prozac, suggesting that the serotonergic system may be involved. "At that point," according to lead author Paul Kenny, "we wanted to know if this increase was behaviorally significant—did it influence the motivation to take the drug?" Evidently it did. **The higher the levels of MeCP2 in the brain, the higher the rats' motivation to consume cocaine.** When the researchers disrupted the expression of MeCP2 with a virus, the rats showed less interest in cocaine.

This is the first evidence that MeCP2 plays some as yet unexplained role in regulating vulnerability to cocaine addiction. **Earlier this summer, investigators reported in *Nature* that another regulatory molecule known as MiRNA-212—a type of RNA involved in gene regulation–had the opposite effect, lessening the test animals' interest in cocaine.** The balancing act between MeCP2 and MiRNA-212 may help explain "the molecular mechanisms that control the transition from controlled to compulsive cocaine intake," according to the paper, although the mechanisms that regulate this balance are not known.

One strong piece of evidence for this regulatory feedback loop was the finding that, while MeCP2 blocked miR-212 expression, the opposite was also true. "We still don't know what exactly influences the activity levels of MeCP2 on miR-212 expression," according to Kenny. **"Now we plan to explore what drives it—whether it's environmentally driven, and if genetic and epigenetic influences are important."**

NIDA director Nora Volkow said in an NIH press release that the work on MeCP2 "exposed an important effect of cocaine at the molecular level that could prove key to understanding compulsive drug taking."

Monday, August 16, 2010

http://addiction-dirkh.blogspot.com/2010/08/chasing-genes-for-cocaine-addiction.html

Im, H., Hollander, J., Bali, P., & Kenny, P. MeCP2 controls BDNF expression and cocaine intake through homeostatic interactions with microRNA-212 *Nature Neuroscience* 2010. DOI: 10.1038/nn.2615

Cannabis Receptors and the "Runner's High"

Maybe it isn't endorphins after all.

What do long-distance running and marijuana smoking have in common? Quite possibly, more than you'd think. A growing body of research suggests that the runner's high and the cannabis high are more similar than previously imagined.

The nature of the runner's high is inconsistent and ephemeral, involving several key neurotransmitters and hormones, and therefore difficult to measure. Much of the evidence comes in the form of animal models. Endocannabinoids—the body's internal cannabis—"seem to contribute to the motivational aspects of voluntary running in rodents." **Knockout mice lacking the cannabinioid CB1 receptor, it turns out, spend less time wheel running than normal mice.**

A Canadian neuroscientist who blogs as NeuroKuz suggests that "a reduction in CB1 levels could lead to less binding of endocannabinoids to receptors in brain circuits that drive motivation to exercise." NeuroKuz speculates on why this might be the case. Physical activity and obtaining rewards are clearly linked. The fittest and fleetest obtain the most food. "A possible explanation for the runner's high, or 'second wind,' a feeling of intense euphoria associated with going on a long run, is that our brains are stuck thinking that lots of exercise should be accompanied by a reward."

In 2004, the *British Journal of Sports Medicine* **ran a research review, "Endocannabinoids and exercise," which seriously disputed the "endorphin hypothesis" assumed to be behind the runner's high.** To begin with, other studies have shown that exercise activates the endocannabinoid system.

"In recent years," according to the authors, "several prominent endorphin researchers—for example, Dr Huda Akil and Dr. Solomon Snyder—have publicly criticised the hypothesis as being 'overly simplistic,' being 'poorly supported by scientific evidence', and a 'myth perpetrated by pop culture.'" **The primary problem is that the opioid system is responsible for respiratory depression, pinpoint pupils, and other effects distinctly unhelpful to runners.**

The investigators wired up college students and put them to work in the gym, and found that "exercise of moderate intensity dramatically increased concentrations of anandamide in blood plasma." The researchers break the runner's high into four major components. Exercise, they say, "suppresses pain, induces sedation, reduces stress, and elevates mood." **Some of the parallels with the cannabis high are not hard to tease out: "Analgesia, sedation (post-exercise calm or glow), a reduction in anxiety, euphoria, and difficulties in estimating the passage of time."**

There are cannabinoid receptors in muscles, skin and the lungs. Intriguingly, the authors suggest that unlike "other rhythmic endurance activities such as swimming, running is a weight bearing sport in which the feet must absorb the 'pounding of the pavement.'" Swimming, the authors speculate, "may not stimulate endocannabinoid release to as great an extent as running." Moreover, "cannabinoids produce neither the respiratory depression, meiosis, or strong inhibition of gastrointestinal motility associated with opiates and opioids. This is because there are few CB1 receptors in the brainstem and, apparently, the large intestine."

A big question remains: **What about running and the "motor inhibition" characteristic of high-dose cannabis?** (An inhibition that may make cannabis useful in the treatment of movement disorders like tremors or tics.) Running a marathon is not the first thing on the minds of most people after getting high on marijuana. The paper maintains, however, that at low doses, "cannabinoids tend to produce hyperactivity," at least in animal models. The CB1 knockout mice were abnormally inactive, due to the effect of cannabinoids on the basal ganglia. Practiced, automatic motor skills like running are controlled in part by the basal ganglia. **The authors predict that "low level skills such as running, which are controlled to a higher degree by the basal ganglia than high level skills, such as basketball, hockey, or tennis, may more readily activate the endocannabinoid system."**

The authors offer other intriguing bits of evidence. Anandamide, one of the brain's own cannabinoids, "acts as a vasodilator and products hypotension, and may thus facilitate blood flow during exercise." In addition, "endocannabinoids and exogenous cannabinoids act as bronchodilators" and could conceivably facilitate breathing during steady exercise. **The authors conclude: "Compared with the opioid analgesics, the analgesia produced by the endocannabinoid system is more consistent with exercise induced analgesia."**

Wednesday, August 4, 2010

http://addiction-dirkh.blogspot.com/2010/08/
cannabis-receptors-and-runners-high.html

Fuss J, Gass P. Endocannabinoids and voluntary activity in mice: runner's high and long-term consequences in emotional behaviors. Experimental Neurology. 224(1):103-5. 2010.

Does Ketamine Cause Bladder Damage?

Special K and cystitis.

Normally, Addiction Inbox steers clear of alarmist stories about drug use. A lifetime of wildly overstated verbiage about "false drugs," as the Firesign Theatre comedy group once delightfully phrased it, has left me wary of drug scare stories. Even obvious cases, like Fetal Alcohol Spectrum Disorder and crack babies, are more nuanced problems than most coverage has alleged.

For years now, rumors about bladder problems in recreational users of ketamine have periodically surfaced. These stories go all the way back to the adventures of Dr. John Lilly, famous for dolphin research, as well as sensory deprivation experiments with LSD, ketamine, and other drugs (wildly overdramatized in the movie, "Altered States"). According to hipster lore, Lilly went through a long period of hourly ketamine ingestion in the 1970s, and ended his days in adult diapers, having lost control of his bladder due to ketamine damage.

To the best of my knowledge, this story has never been officially confirmed. But in the last two years, research has surfaced that tends to bolster the Lilly anecdote. What is disturbing is that today, unlike 40 years ago, ketamine has become a fairly common party drug among young users. The drug technically produces a state of "dissociative anesthesia." Treated like a hallucinogen, ketamine was originally a tranquilizer used in veterinary medicine. In 1970, the

FDA approved the use of ketamine for humans for the maintenance of anesthesia. It is now being tested for use in PTSD and intractable depression.

The journey from horse tranquilizer to party drug has eluded drug researchers until quite recently. However, in early 2008, researchers sat up and took notice of a report published in *BJU International*, a urology journal: "The destruction of the lower urinary tract by ketamine abuse: a new syndrome?"

The report details the discovery by physicians in Hong Kong of 59 ketamine abusers who had been admitted to urology units in local hospitals from 2000 to 2007. Interstitial cystitis, also known as painful bladder syndrome, can vary from mild to severe, and its cause is often not known. Symptoms include painful, frequent, or urgent urination. The researchers found that 71 % of the patients "showed various degrees of epithelial inflammation similar to that seen in chronic interstitial cystitis. All of 12 available bladder biopsies had histological features resembling those of interstitial cystitis."

The authors conclude that "secondary renal damage can occur in severe cases, which might be irreversible, rendering patients dependent on dialysis."

Scary stuff. If this were the only study available, it would be tempting to question the results. As it turns out, the Hong Kong study was neither the first nor the last. What is believed to be the first official report of the problem appeared in 2007 in *Urology*, documenting the case of nine Canadian ketamine users with bladder complications. The authors, affiliated with the University of Toronto, conclude: **"As illicit ketamine becomes more easily available, ulcerative cystitis and potential long-term bladder sequelae related to its use may be a more prevalent problem confronting urologists."**

This year, similar reports from Bristol in the UK were published in *Clinical Radiology*. Researchers with the National Health Service and the Bristol Royal Infirmary discovered "a series of 23 patients, all with a history of ketamine abuse, who presented with severe lower urinary tract symptoms." **Various imaging techniques revealed smaller bladder volume, bladder wall thickening, inflammation, urethral strictures, and other bladder pathologies.** The patients all reported symptoms similar to those reported by the earlier Hong Kong ketamine users.

The report concludes that "many users are well aware, but are often not forthcoming with this information." They also maintain that "the key to the effective management of ketamine-induced bladder pathology is early diagnosis."

Frequent recreational use of ketamine appears ill advised until more research can confirm the true scope of the problem.

Thursday, October 21, 2010

http://addiction-dirkh.blogspot.com/2010/10/does-ketamine-cause-bladder-damage.html

Chu, P., Ma, W., Wong, S., Chu, R., Cheng, C., Wong, S., Tse, J., Lau, F., Yiu, M., & Man, C. The destruction of the lower urinary tract by ketamine abuse: a new syndrome? *BJU International, 102* (11), 1616-1622. 2008. DOI: 10.1111/j.1464-410X.2008.07920.x

Era of the Electronic Cigarette Officially Begins

Court blocks FDA from prohibiting e-cigarettes.

It's official: The e-cigarette is here. The right of a distributor of Chinese electronic cigarettes to market the product in the U.S. was solidly affirmed last week by a three-judge ruling in the U.S. Court of Appeals for the District of Columbia. The Food and Drug Administration's refusal last year to allow importation of e-cigarettes by Sottera Inc. had been the basis for a lower court decision in Sottera's favor. The earlier court ruled that e-cigarettes did not require FDA approval because they were neither new drugs nor new drug delivery devices. (The FDA is prohibited by an act of Congress from barring the sale of tobacco products outright.)

Last month, under a consent judgement worked out with California state Attorney General Jerry Brown in a related case, Florida-based Smoking Everywhere Co., another distributor of Chinese electronic cigarettes, had agreed not to target minors in its advertising, or to make claims that its products are safe alternatives to tobacco. The move came shortly after the FDA announced plans to regulate battery-powered e-cigarettes as new drug delivery devices, culminating in the Sottera lawsuit.

The legal argument before the appeals court hinged largely on semantics. The court found that electronic cigarettes are "battery-powered products that allow users to inhale nicotine vapor without fire, smoke, ash or carbon monoxide. The liquid nic-otine is derived from natural tobacco plants."

Here is the catch: "The FDA may only approve a product for marketing under the Federal Food, Drug and Cosmetic Act (FDCA) if it is safe and effective for its intended use," the Appeals Court Justices ruled. However, the FDA has "exhaustively documented" that tobacco products are unsafe for pharmacological use of any kind. The earlier court had concluded, stealing a page from "Alice in Wonderland": **"If they cannot be used safely for any thera-peutic purpose, and yet they cannot be banned, they sim-ply do not fit"** within any conceivable regulatory scheme.

Hence the difficulties in the FDA's attempt to regulate by agency fiat. E-cigarette manufacturers and distributors, having sensed an opening, are now ready to drive a convoy of semis right through it. This wasn't a completely straightforward march, as the e-ciga-rette forces, in the appeals presentation, were required to thread the needle on such conundrums as: Does it matter that e-cigarettes do not, strictly speaking, contain "tobacco products?" Nicotine is a component of, not a product of, tobacco.

You see the problem. **The relevant statutes have not been written with pure nicotine delivery devices in mind.** In fact, having nicotine—but not the evil substance tobacco—in your product turned out to be a definitional advantage for the e-cigarette marketers: The court pointed out that, unlike products containing tobacco, which the FDA has found to be associated with "cancer, respiratory illnesses, and heart disease," the FDA has manifestly *not* found that nicotine or tobacco-free products that deliver nicotine are inherently unsafe. And second, the "tobacco-specific legislation" invoked in earlier court cases "simply does not address products that deliver nicotine but contain no tobacco."

Matthew Myers, president of the Campaign for Tobacco-Free Kids, said in a prepared statement: **"This decision will allow** any manufacturer to put any level of nicotine in any product and sell it to anybody, including children, with no government regulation or oversight at the present time. We urge the government to appeal this ruling."

Among the many questions the ruling leaves open is the status of e-cigarettes under existing no-smoking regulations. That litigation has not even gotten underway.

Thursday, December 9, 2010

http://addiction-dirkh.blogspot.com/2010/12/
era-of-electronic-cigarette-officially.html

Consider the CB(2) Receptor

A different destination for cannabinoids.

THC and its organic cousin, anandamide, do what they do by locking into both the CB1 receptor, discovered in 1988, and the CB2 receptor (as it is commonly written in shorthand), discovered 5 years later. THC and anandamide are CB receptor agonists, meaning they activate the receptors in question. (An antagonist blocks the receptor's action.)

CB1 is a very common receptor in the central nervous system, and, when stimulated by an agonist, is responsible for the well-known roster of alleged medical effects, such as pain relief and nausea from chemotherapy—along with the typical marijuana high. (For more on this, see the excellent 2007 post by Dr. Joan Bushwell.) **Conversely, blocking CB1 activity with an antagonist like rimonabant is one controversial avenue being explored in the search for new weight loss drugs.** (CB1 antagonists can also produce anxiety and depression.)

However, CB2 was long considered a "peripheral" cannabinoid receptor, meaning that scientists hadn't managed to find CB2 receptors in the central nervous system. They were, however, plentiful in the immune system, and seemed to be involved in inflammation as well as pain responses. **CB2 receptors were in fact eventually discovered in the central nervous system, and are**

active in the brain during certain kinds of inflammatory responses.

There is a straightforward commercial incentive for tracking the extent of CB2 expression in brain neurons. As the authors of a cannabinoid receptor study wrote in the June issue of the *British Journal of Pharmacology:*

"As CB(2) is an attractive therapeutic target for pain management and immune system modulation without overt psychoactivity, defining the extent of its presence in neurons will have a significant impact on drug discovery."

Translated, this means that there are a number of new molecules that are selective for CB2 receptors. Since people don't get a strong traditional marijuana-style buzz from CB2 receptor activation, and given the active involvement of CB2 receptors in things like immune responses and inflammatory reactions, the possibility exists of finding lucrative spinoffs like pain pills or anti-inflammatory medications. So drug researchers would like to know exactly where those receptors are, and what they do, in the event that they end up attempting to make a medicine that stimulates or blocks them artificially. (Credit to Vaughan Bell of Mind Hacks for highlighting this study.)

The psychologists at Indiana University who produced the paper did their best to shed light on where the CB(2) receptor is hiding, and what, exactly, it does. But there is still not enough known about how various substances react with this somewhat elusive receptor for cannabinoids. **In 2008, scientists at the University of Madrid published research in the *Journal of Biological Chemistry* indicating that activation of the CB2 receptor reduced nerve cell loss in animals suffering from a disease similar to multiple sclerosis.** Researchers point to the possibility that a safe drug for M.S. patients could be one of the results of CB2 research.

Thursday, July 8, 2010

http://addiction-dirkh.blogspot.com/2010/07/consider-cb2-receptor.html

Atwood, B., & Mackie, K. CB2: a cannabinoid receptor with an identity crisis British Journal of Pharmacology, 160 (3), 467-479. 2010. DOI: 10.1111/j.1476-5381.2010.00729.x

Cancer and Women Who Drink: A Flawed Study?

Taking a second look at the numbers.

A recent front page *Washington Post* story on the increased risk of cancer among women who drink shed more heat than light on the underlying conundrum: Are a few drinks good for you, or aren't they?

A British study involving almost one and a quarter million women—a huge survey by any standards—found that just one drink of alcohol per day increased the statistical risk of contracting cancer. According to the *Post* story by Rob Stein, as little as 10 grams of alcohol a day elevated women's risk for cancer of the breast, liver, and rectum in particular. "Based on the findings, the researchers estimated that about 5 percent of all cancers diagnosed in women each year in the United States are the result of low to moderate alcohol consumption," the *Post* reported. "Most are breast cancers, with drinking accounting for 11 percent of cases—about 20,000 extra cases each year—the researchers estimated."

But wait a minute. **Wasn't it just yesterday that researchers were confirming and reconfirming that a couple of drinks a day was good for your heart?** Presumably, this included women's hearts as well. What's going on?

For starters, the conclusions of the study itself, published in the *Journal of the National Cancer Institute*, have some problems. In an article entitled, "Women: How Bad is a Regular Nip?" Janet Raloff writes in the Web edition of *Science News* that female participants were queried only about *weekly* alcohol consumption. **To arrive at figures for daily intake, the researchers divided by seven.** "However," writes Raloff, "if someone averages seven drinks a week, those beverages might have been downed on weekends only—leading to consumption of three or more drinks at a sitting. That would be bad even for the heart. Also, in the long haul, for anyone's liver." Unless we know about daily drinking, the study "only offers fodder for speculation."

There are other problems. **As it turns out, *nondrinkers* have an elevated risk for certain kinds of cancers**. Study author Naomi Allen and coworkers at the University of Oxford write that alcohol apparently confers some sort of protective effect when it comes to cancers of the pharynx, esophagus, stomach, cervix, and other sites.

In addition, Raloff, points out, "There's the impact of smoking." **Some of the alcohol-linked cases of cancer in women—esophagus, liver, and larynx, for example—increased only among those women in the study who also smoked.**

Specifically, Raloff recommends that women with a genetic predisposition for breast cancer might decide that "no alcohol is the best policy." And for people at low risk for heart disease, it's difficult to justify drinking because it's good for your heart. However, "study after study has offered quantitative evidence that middle-age and older adults who take a regular nip—like that proverbial glass of sherry after dinner or at bedtime—suffer less heart disease and diabetes than teetotalers or people who consume more than two drinks a day."

And that, at present, is where the matter still stands. As Raloff sensibly concludes, "Let's not scare people with incomplete data.

There will be plenty of time to hammer home a call for temperance if and when stronger data emerge."

Monday, March 2, 2009

http://addiction-dirkh.blogspot.com/2009/03/
cancer-and-women-who-drink-flawed-study.html

What's a Neurotransmitter, Anyway?

A brief guide for the perplexed.

A neurotransmitter is a chemical substance that carries impulses from one nerve cell to another. Neurotransmitters are manufactured by the body and are released from storage sacs in the nerve cells. A tiny junction, called the synaptic gap, lies between brain cells. (Think of Michelangelo's Sistine Chapel, with the finger of Adam and the finger of God not quite touching, yet conveying energy and information.)

Neurotransmitters squirt across the synaptic gap, and this shower of chemical messengers lands on a field of tiny bumps attached to the surface of the nerve cell on the other side of the synaptic gap. These bumps are receptors, and they have distinctive shapes. Picture these receptors, brain researcher Candace Pert has suggested, as a field of lily pads floating on the outer oily surface of the cell.

Neurotransmitter molecules bind themselves tightly to these receptors. The fact that certain drugs of abuse also lock tightly into existing receptors, and send messages to nerve cells in the brain, is the key to the mystery of addiction.

The fact that certain drugs essentially "fool" receptors into receiving them is one of the most important and far-reaching discoveries in the history of modern science. It is the reason why even minute amounts of certain drugs can have such powerful effects on the human nervous system. The lock-and-key arrangement of neurotransmitters and their receptors is the fundamental architecture of action in the brain. Glandular cells are studded with receptors, and many of the hormones have their own receptors as well. If the drug fits the receptor and elicits a response, it is called an agonist. If it simply blocks the receptor site without stimulating a response, it is an antagonist. Still other neurotransmitters have only a secondary effect, causing the target cell to release other kinds of neurotransmitters and hormones.

Two of the most important neurotransmitters are serotonin and dopamine. The unfolding story of addiction science, at bottom, is the story of what has been learned about the nature and function of such chemicals, and the many and varied ways they effect the pleasure and reward centers in our brains.

In 1948, three researchers—Maurice Rapport, Arda Green, and Irvine Page—were looking for a better blood pressure medication. Instead, they managed to isolate a naturally occurring compound in beef blood called serotonin (pronounced sarah-tóne-in), and known chemically as 5-hydroxytryptamine, or simply 5-HT. The researchers determined that serotonin was involved in vasoconstriction, or narrowing of the blood vessels, and in that respect resembled another important chemical messenger in the brain—epinephrine, better known as adrenaline.

Even though there is at most 10 milligrams of the substance in our bodies, serotonin turned out to be one of nature's signature chemicals—a chemical of thought, movement and behavior, as well as digestion, ejaculation, and evacuation. The body's all-purpose neurotransmitter, involved in sleep, mood, appetite, among dozens of other functions. **The cortex, the limbic system, the brain stem, the gut, the genitals, the bowels: serotonin is a key chemical messenger in all of it.**

Another key neurotransmitter—dopamine—is considered to be one of the brain's primary "pleasure chemicals," and is found in areas of the brain linked to experiences of joy and reward.

Dopamine pathways play a role in carrying signals related to attention, movement, problem solving, pleasure, and the anticipation of rewarding experiences. Dopamine is one of the reasons why, after you have a pleasurable experience with food, drink, sex, or certain drugs, you are likely to feel a desire to repeat the experience. **Dopamine is implicated in not just the drug high, but in the craving that accompanies withdrawal as well.**

Feelings of pleasure, or joy, are natural drug highs. The fact that they are produced by chemical alterations in brain state does not make the fear or the pleasure feel any less real.

Tuesday, July 7, 2009

http://addiction-dirkh.blogspot.com/2009/07/whats-neurotransmitter-anyway.html

2) The New Synthetics

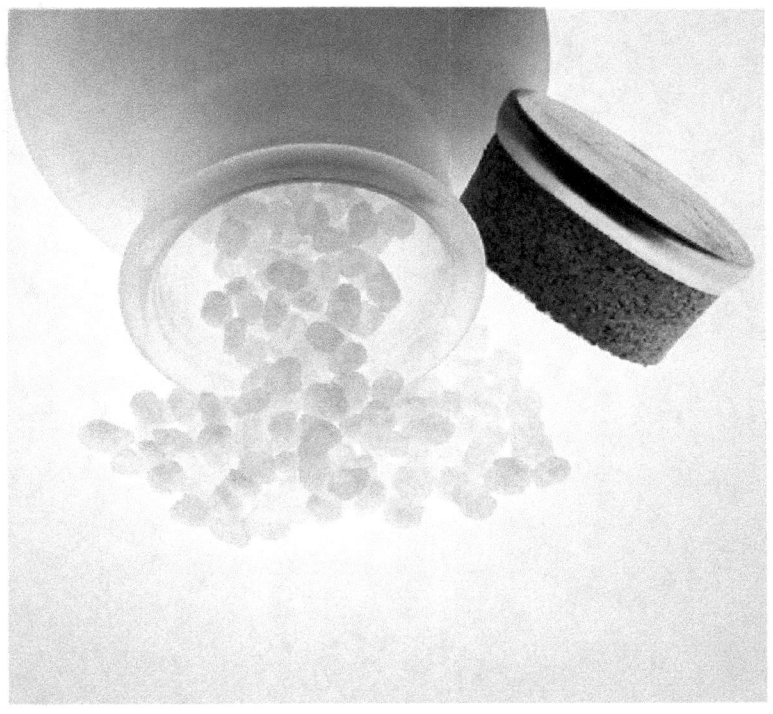

(National Institute of Drug Abuse)

Mephedrone, the New Drug in Town

Bull market for quasi-legal designer highs.

Most people in the United States have never heard of it. Very few have ever tried it. But if Europe is any kind of leading indicator for synthetic drugs (and it is), then America in 2010 will have a chance to get acquainted with mephedrone, a.k.a. Drone, MCAT, 4-methylmethcathinone (4-MMC), and Meow Meow—the latter nickname presumably in honor of its membership in the cathinone family, making it chemically similar in some ways to amphetamine and ephedrine. But its users often refer to effects more commonly associated with Ecstasy (MDMA), both the good (euphoria, empathy, talkativeness) and the bad (blood pressure spikes, delusions, drastic changes in body temperature).

Some of the best stateside coverage has come from the anonymous NIH researcher who blogs on science topics as DrugMonkey. The whole business of what mephedrone does is complicated, he writes. **The cathinone structure is "very similar to amphetamine and supports parallel modifications," but there is clearly an "MDMA-like component to this mephedrone stuff."**

Until earlier this year, mephedrone was in that weird state of limbo LSD found itself occupying in the mid-1960s: legal, but not for long. States are attempting to sweep synthetic drugs of abuse like Spice and other cannabinioid derivatives into a proscribed package that includes mephedrone. **Federal authorities are able to prosecute under The Analogue Drug Act of 1986, which was designed to combat this dilemma in the United States by outlawing drugs "substantially similar" to any drug that is already illegal.** However, "chemical experts disagree on whether a chemical is 'substantially similar' in structure to another chemical—so much so that Federal Analogue Act litigation often degenerates into a 'battle of experts,' which is founded more on opinion than on actual scientific evidence," writes Gregory Kau in an article for the *University of Pennsylvania Law Review.*

It is clear by now that this cat-and-mouse game is rigged in favor of the designers and suppliers of new drugs under the sun. Exploiting the gray zone of quasi-legality is extremely profitable. **One outlaw chemist told Jeanne Whalen of the *Wall Street Journal* that by the time law enforcement closes in, "we are going to bring out something else."** At which point, prosecutorial mechanisms put in place for mephedrone must be laboriously recreated for the new drug.

This drug entrepreneur, and others like him, makes extensive use of the Internet, especially in Europe, since mephedrone is not universally banned. **To keep the business technically legal, sellers label mephedrone "not for human consumption" and market it as anything from plant food to bath salts.** Sometimes they draw unwanted attention to themselves through the purchase of lab equipment.

Mephedrone has lately been covered relentlessly by the British press, after the deaths of three young people in the U.K. and Sweden were attributed to mephedrone. Part of the difficulty in assessing the danger and addictiveness, if any, of these newer substances is that most of them have not been subjected to controlled clinical testing on humans. (One hardy purveyor of mephedrone snorted half a gram of the drug on a Belgian news program to demonstrate his side of the argument.)

Media hysteria in the U.K. led to reports of dozens of deaths due to mephedrone. As British politicians rushed to enact a ban, Danny Kushlick of the drug charity Transform told the *U.K. Guardian* in April: **"The misreporting of mephedrone deaths is a crass example of the potentially lethal alliance between press and politicians that by default ends in a ban that often creates far greater harms than those caused by use."** In July, BBC News reported that the mephedrone crackdown was "floundering", even though the ban had been widened to included a near-beer version of mephedrone called Naphyrone (sold as NRG1). But a spokesperson for Lifeline, another British drug charity, argued that "you can't just ban your way out of a problem because it could result in far more dangerous chemicals coming onto the market." According to the European Monitoring Centre for Drugs and Drug Addiction, which operates the EU early-warning system on new drugs in cooperation with Europol, "24 new psychoactive substances were officially notified for the first time to the two agencies in 2009."

The National Drug Intelligence Center at the U.S. Department of Justice reported that early in the year, "several individuals in the Bismarck [North Dakota] area ingested or injected illicit products containing mephedrone and required hospitalization. In addition, the Oregon State Police Forensic Laboratory (Bend, Oregon) received two submission of white power that users referred to as 'sunshine.' Both submissions tested as mephedrone."

And now comes a report from North Carolina of two fatalities allegedly linked to the use of mephedrone, as reported by David Kroll at Terra Sigillata.

Narcotics officials and toxicologists say that the raw materials for many of the new drugs appear to be manufactured in China and trans-shipped to other countries in Southeast Asia and the Middle East. DrugMonkey also notes that it will be interesting to see "if actions such as Cambodia, Vietnam, and Thailand finally getting serious about controlling the production of the safrole oil used as a precursor in MDMA manufacture is having a lasting effect on world markets."

Tuesday, November 2, 2010

http://addiction-dirkh.blogspot.com/2010/11/mephedrone-new-drug-in-town.html

Tracking Synthetic Highs

UN office monitors designer drug trade.

Produced by the United Nations Office on Drugs and Crime (UNODC), the Global SMART Update for October 2010 provides interim reports of emerging trends in synthetic drug use. The report does not concern itself with cocaine, heroin, marijuana, alcohol, or tobacco. "Unlike plant-based drugs," says the report, "synthetic drugs are quickly evolving with new designer drugs appearing on the market each year." The update deals primarily with amphetamine-type stimulants, but also includes newer designer drugs such as mephedrone, atypical synthetics like ketamine, synthetic opioids like fentanyl, and old standbys like LSD.

I have summarized some of the findings below:

The first methamphetamine lab in 15 years has been discovered in Japan. Japanese law enforcement seized a suspected residential methamphetamine laboratory outside of Tokyo, the first such seizure since 1995. Two Iranian nationals were arrested. Given the continuously high price of imported crystalline methamphetamine in Japan, there is an increased likelihood that more domestic manufacturers could emerge.

Record ketamine seizures and use has been reported by Taiwan province of China. The FDA reports that ketamine seizures in the first five months of 2010 alone totaled 1465 KG, nearly 300 KG more than last year. Concurrent increases in use were also noted.

The first methamphetamine laboratory in Turkey was discovered. Local media reported the seizure of the lab, in the southern part of the country. The facility reportedly planned to manufacture 100,000 tablets for retail sale at USD 13.40 apiece. In 2009, Turkey reported its first seizures of methamphetamine totaling 103 KG at Istanbul's airport, which has become a transit point for methamphetamine traffic from Iran to markets in East Asia.

Law enforcement faces unique challenges when dealing with synthetic drug analogs. Customs officers at Prague's Ruzyne airport reported arresting a Polish national for transporting a substance initially testing positive for ephedrone, a controlled synthetic stimulant. Confirmatory tests, however, revealed the substance to be mephedrone, an analogue not under international control. The event illustrates the challenges law enforcement face when encountering new synthetic substances not under national or international control.

Amphetamine breathalyzer tests may soon be possible, say Swedish researchers. The June issue of the *Journal of Analytical Toxicology* reported that the first breath test for methamphetamine and amphetamine detection was successfully conducted in Sweden. Drugs in the exhaled breath are captured in a filter and analyzed using a combination of liquid chromatography and mass spectrometry. Experimental trials on amphetamine-dependent patients admitted to hospital urgency rooms for overdose provided the same results as traditional drug tests.

The U.S. is expanding controls on precursor chemicals for fentanyl and LSD. The Drug Enforcement Administration (DEA) has designated a compound called ANPP as a precursor chemical for fentanyl, an extremely potent synthetic analgesic. Earlier this year, the DEA proposed new controls over ergocristine, a chemical precursor sometimes used in the manufacture of LSD. Clandestine laboratories in the United States employ it as a substitute for ergotamine and ergometrine, both of which are already under international control.

The U.S. indicts 15 people in one of the largest MDMA busts ever. The U.S. Department of Justice announced that a federal grand jury indicted 15 men linked to one of the country's largest ecstasy manufacturing and trafficking rings. Two storage facilities were also seized during the investigation, yielding about 710,000 MDMA tablets. Law enforcement authorities seized more than 1.1 million tablets in all. Authorities believe that the group had been responsible for the distribution of hundreds of thousands of MDMA tablets each month.

Belize stops large shipments of methamphetamine precursors bound for Mexico. Customs authorities in Belize reportedly stopped two large shipments of phenylacetic acid (PAA), or roughly 46 metric tons. Phenylacetic acid can be used in the manufacture of methamphetamine. Reports suggest the chemical came from China and was ultimately destined for Mexico.

Friday, October 29, 2010

http://addiction-dirkh.blogspot.com/2010/10/tracking-synthetic-highs.html

Marijuana: The New Generation

What's in that "Spice" packet?

They first turned up in Europe and the U.K.; those neon-colored foil packets labeled "Spice," sold in small stores and novelty shops, next to the 2 oz. power drinks and the caffeine pills. Unlike the stimulants known as mephedrone or M-Cat, or the several variations on the formula for MDMA—both of which have also been marketed as Spice and "bath salts"—the bulk of the new products in the Spice line were synthetic versions of cannabis.

The new forms of synthetic cannabis tickle the same brain receptors as THC does, and are sometimes capable of producing feelings of well-being, empathy, and euphoria—in other words, pretty much the same effects that draw people to pot. But along the way, users began turning up in the emergency room, something that very rarely happens in the case of smoked marijuana. The symptoms were similar to adverse effects some people experience with marijuana, but greatly exaggerated: extreme anxiety and paranoia, and heart palpitations.

As it turns out, there is a very real difference between smoking Purple Kush and snorting "Banana Cream Nuke" out of a metallic packet. **The difference lies in the manner in which the brain's receptors for cannabinoids are stimulated by the new cannabis compounds.** When things goes wrong at the CB1 and CB2 receptors, and the mix isn't right, the results may not be euphoria, giggles, short-term memory loss, and the munchies, but rather "nausea, anxiety, agitation/panic attacks, tachycardia, paranoid ideation, and hallucinations." Furthermore, the Spice variants do not contain cannabidiol, a cannabis ingredient that has been shown to reduce anxiety in animal models, and reduces THC-induced anxiety in human volunteers. The authors of a recent study suggest that the "lack of this cannabinoid in Spice drugs may exacerbate the detrimental effects of these herbal mixtures on emotion and sociability."

What concerned the researchers was that, in addition to reports of cognitive deficits and emotional alterations and gastrointestinal effects, emergency room physicians were reporting wildly elevated heart rates, extremely high blood pressure, chest pains, and fever. **Fattore and Fratta report that "two adolescents died in the USA after ingestion of a Spice product called 'K2,'" one due to a coronary ischemic event, and the other due to suicide.** What's going on?

In a paper for *Frontiers in Behavioral Neuroscience* called "Beyond THC: the new generation of cannabinoid designer drugs," Liana Fattore and Walter Fratta of the University Of Cagliari in Monserrato, Italy, identified more than 140 different products marketed as Spice, and laid out the extreme variability found in composition and potency. **Like a mutating virus, they came to the U.S., starting in early 2009, a new strain seemingly every week: Spice, K2, Spice Gold, Silver, Arctic Spice, Genie, Dream, and dozens of others, the naming and renaming suggesting nothing so much as the proliferating strains of high-end marijuana: Skunk, Haze, Silver Haze, Amnesia, AK-47.** Synthetic marijuana comes mainly from manufacturers in Asia, and second generation chemicals have already been put on a to-be-banned list by the DEA. States have jumped all over the problem with duplicate legislation, despite the fact that experts believe a majority of sales take place over the Internet. A third generation of synthetic cannabis variants, which are sprinkled on an herbal base and meant to be snorted, are openly sold and touted as legal. And they *are* legal, depending upon which one you buy, and where you buy it. **Synthetic cannabis is still readily available, affordably packaged, and right on the shelf, or ready for purchase online—unlike the frequently vague and sometimes shady process of scoring a bag of weed**. In the beginning, at least, the new drugs were perceived by youthful users as safer than other drugs.

But the most crucial attribute of Spice and related products is that they are not detectable in urine and blood samples. You can cruise all night on Spice, and test clean the next day at work. The kind of cannabis in Spice doesn't read out on anybody's drug tests as marijuana. That requires the presence of THC—and the new synthetics don't have any.

There are four different categories of chemicals used in the manufacture of "cannabimimetic" drugs. The first and best known is the so-called JWH series of "novel cannabinoids" synthesized by John W. Huffman at Clemson University in the 1980s. The most widely used variant is an extremely potent version known as JWH-018. While JWH-018 is, chemically speaking, not structurally like THC at all, it snaps onto CB1 and CB2 receptors more fiercely than THC itself. The CP-compounds, the second class of synthetic compounds, were developed back in the 1970s by Pfizer, when that firm was actively engaged in testing cannabis-like compounds for commercial potential, a program they later dropped. The best-known example is CP-47,497. While CP-47,497 lacks the chemical structure of classic cannabinoids, it is anywhere from 3 to 28 times more potent than THC, and shows classic THC-like effects in animal studies. The next group is known as HU-compounds, because they originated at Hebrew University, where much of the early work on the mechanisms of THC took place. The last category consists of chemicals in the family of benzoylindoles, which also show an affinity for cannabinoid receptors.

JWH-018, the most common form of synthetic cannabis, and now widely illegal, is considerably more potent than THC—4 times stronger at the CB1 receptor, and 10 times stronger at the less familiar CB2 receptor. The CB2 receptor seems to have a lot to do with pain perception and inflammation, which is why researchers continue to investigate it. **But CB2 receptors contribute only indirectly to the classic marijuana high, which is all about THC's affinity for CB1 receptors, and the effects of using drugs with a very strong affinity for CB2 receptors is not well documented.** And therein might lie the source of the problem—or, as Fattore and Fratta describe it, "the greater prevalence of adverse effects observed with JWH-018-containing products relative to marijuana." A popular compound of the second kind, HU-210, has frequently been found in herbal mixtures available in the U.S. and U.K. According to the study, "the pharmacological effects of HU-210 in vivo are also exceptionally long lasting, and in animal models it has been shown to negatively affect learning and memory processes as well as sexual behavior."

That, in a nutshell, is what the kids are smoking these days. But wait, there's more: **Besides synthetic cannabinoids, herbs and vitamins, researchers have found opioids like tramadol, opioid receptor-active compounds like Kratom (Mitragyna speciosa), and oleamide, a fatty acid derivative with psychoactive properties. (A combination of oleamide and JWH-018 has been sold as "Aroma.")** Indentifying which of these active ingredients is part of any particular packet of "legal highs" is further complicated by manufacturers' tendency to mix the ingredients together with various organic compounds—everything from nicotine to masking agents like vitamin E. In fact, almost anything that might make it more difficult for forensic labs to pry it all apart: alfalfa, comfrey leaf, passionflower, horehound, etc. Banana Cream Nuke, which was purchased in an American smoke shop, and made two young girls very sick, contained 15 varieties of synthetic cannabis—but none of the herbal ingredients actually listed on the label.

Unlike the partial activation of CB1 receptors by THC, which takes place when people smoke marijuana, "synthetic cannabinoids identified so far in Spice products have been shown to act as full agonists with increased potency, thus leading to longer durations of action and an increased likelihood of adverse effects." When it comes to cannabis, users are far better off smoking the real thing, from a harm reduction standpoint, and staying clear of these unpredictable synthetic substitutes.

Wednesday, November 2, 2011

http://addiction-dirkh.blogspot.com/2011/11/marijuana-new-generation.html

Fattore, L., & Fratta, W. Beyond THC: The New Generation of Cannabinoid Designer Drugs *Frontiers in Behavioral Neuroscience, 5* 2011. DOI: 10.3389/fnbeh.2011.00060

MDMA Likes It Hot

X and ambient air temperature.

One of the enduring mysteries about MDMA, the popular amphetamine derivative known as Ecstasy, or X, is the relationship between the drug and ambient air temperature. Why are raves hot, sweaty, and full of loud music and flashing lights? Because "human subjects report a higher euphoric state when taking the drug in sensory rich environments," according to researchers. So there's a reason for all those glow sticks and speaker stacks. But is it something inherent in the mechanism of the drug—or simply the overheated party atmosphere combined with vigorous dancing—that can sometimes raise a ravers' body temperature to dangerous levels?

Drug researchers have known for some time that Ecstasy and high temperature are somehow interlinked. **Animal studies have produced strong evidence that a heated environment can cause an increase in MDMA-stimulated serotonin 5-HT response. Many ravers take steps to prevent hyperthermia, or overheating, by regularly drinking water and coming off the dance floor at regular intervals**. Most people have heard of hypothermia, a condition in which body temperature drops to dangerously low levels. But hyperthermia can be just as deadly, and it is a common emergency room complaint in MDMA admissions.

In animal models, rats on MDMA (they like it enough to self-administer) show significantly elevated responses to serotonin in the nucleus accumbens at high room temperatures. What does that mean? What goes up must come down: It opens the door to possible serotonin depletion, which can cause dysfunctions in mood and cognition. Researchers at the University of Texas in Austin have found that in rodents, "the magnitude of the hyperthermic response has been tightly correlated with MDMA-induced 5-HT depletion in various brain regions." **The question they pose is whether "elevated ambient temperatures, such as those encountered in rave venues, can exacerbate MDMA-induced temperature-increasing effects and the likelihood of adverse drug effects."** (Cocaine has temperature-related effects as well. When the ambient air temperature is higher than 75 degrees F, accidental cocaine overdoses increase.)

Ecstasy boosts dopamine as well. The Texas researchers suggest that "the combined enhancement of 5-HT and dopamine may contribute to MDMA's unique effects on thermoregulation." **They also found that core temperature responses appeared to be "experience-dependent," meaning that rats didn't show significantly elevated core temperatures in warm rooms until after they had rolled with MDMA at least ten times.** And the worse it gets, the worse it gets, according to the report, published in *European Neuropsychopharmacology*: "Our results suggest that a heated environment facilitates MDMA-induced disruption of homeostatic thermoregulatory responses, but that repeated exposure to MDMA may also disrupt thermoregulation regardless of ambient temperature."

So, while all that sweaty dancing amps up the perceptual effects of Ecstasy, it isn't necessarily implicated in overheating. To simulate a nightclub full of X-ed out ravers, investigators at the Scripps Research Institute tested rats on MDMA while the animals exercised on activity wheels. **Writing in *Pharmacology Biochemistry and Behavior*, the researchers found that "wheel activity did**

not modify the hyperthermia produced.... These results suggest that nightclub dancing in the human Ecstasy consumer may not be a significant factor in medical emergencies."

Bottom line: Although we have a reasonable idea of how it works in animals, we don't really know how much of that knowledge applies to humans in rave settings. Research aimed at teasing out the specifics of temperature-related responses to MDMA is ongoing. And it does matter. Frequent heat-induced responses could lead to prolonged 5-HT depletion, which is suspected of causing an escalation of drug intake in experienced Ecstasy users. And frequent, escalating use of MDMA is implicated in a long roster of potential cognitive impairments.

Wednesday, March 28, 2012

http://addiction-dirkh.blogspot.com/2012/03/mdma-likes-it-hot.html

The Low Down on
the New Highs

Not all bath salts are alike.

You're 16 hours into your 24-hour shift on the medic unit, and you find yourself responding to an "unknown problem" call....Walking up to the patient, you note a slender male sitting wide-eyed on the sidewalk. His skin is noticeably flushed and diaphoretic, and he appears extremely tense.You notice slight tremors in his upper body, a clenched jaw and a vacant look in his eyes....As you begin to apply the blood pressure cuff, the patient begins violently resisting and thrashing about on the sidewalk—still handcuffed. Nothing seems to calm him, and he simultaneously bangs his head on the sidewalk and tries to kick you... and his body temperature is 103.2° F. He doesn't respond with anything other than basic "yes" and "no" answers. Recognizing the probable state of acute stimulant intoxication and the risks associated, you begin further treatment.You turn the patient compartment air conditioning on high and obtain large-bore IV access of normal saline and set an initial infusion rate of 250 cc/hour.... Later in your shift, you return to the same emergency department (ED) and are informed that the patient has been admitted for rhabdomyolysis and has admitted to taking "bath salts" for the past three days."

This episode, taken from an article in a recent issue of the *Journal of Emergency Medical Services* by Jon Nevin, a California emergency medical technician and paramedic, aptly demonstrates the dilemmas facing medical workers since the explosion in usage of "bath salts." A catchall category for a family of designer stimulants centered on chemicals known as cathinones, bath salts, which are of course no such thing, began filtering in from Europe. One of the more popular new club drugs was variously called meph, or CAT, or 4-MMC, or Meow Meow. The drug's official name was mephedrone. It was a chemical cousin of amphetamine, with effects somewhat similar to those of Ecstasy (MDMA).

In 2011, calls to poison controls centers skyrocketed across the country as new and untested combinations of cathinones came on the market. Bewildered emergency room technicians and toxicologists were hard pressed to identify even basic ingredients. **Recreational users never knew what was in the shiny foil packages, only what was purportedly *not* in them—a laundry list of recently proscribed chemicals, which the marketers proudly noted on the packaging.** This endless Mobius strip of designer stimulant development and grey-market sales channels mean a lucrative hit-and-run business for the producers, but a completely unsafe landscape for recreational users, who act as voluntary guinea pigs for new combinations of poorly understood psychoactive compounds. It is from this underground designer milieu that MDMA came to the forefront, courtesy of clandestine work done by neurochemist Alexander Shulgin and associates.

Mephedrone started showing up in the U.S. in 2010, and quickly spread via word of mouth and the Internet. This was not the synthetic marijuana in powder form being marketed as Spice and K2, although distribution channels were often the same. This was synthetic speed that could be dissolved and injected. **The idea was, you could get high and still pass a random drug test, since drug tests didn't have the sophisticated assays needed to sort out the cathinones.** And you could escape the tightening net around Ecstasy use, and still get Ecstasy-like effects. And designer stimulants picked up another strong user base: heroin addicts and methadone users looked for a detection-free boost. They could stay enrolled in their methadone program, and dodge trouble with parole officers, and still party all weekend on bath salts. **One big problem became apparent straightaway: The effect of bath salts varied wildly, from gentle stimulant to some sort of death's-head equivalent of the brown acid at Woodstock.**

Bath salts were easy to buy. These unregulated stimulants came in a bewildering array of mixtures, featuring dozens of ingredients and additives. Even when they weren't blatantly available on the shelves of head shops and convenience stores, many outlets carried them—if you knew the street codes. What law enforcement officer would bust you for buying jewelry cleaner, for example? Cops and drug enforcement officers must long for the clarity of the old days. You had smack, you had crack, you had bathtub Methedrine (methamphetamine).

"Understanding what each of those substances can do physiologically is key to understanding their dangers and to determining how best to treat people who need medical assistance," wrote Marc Kaufman, with the McLean Imaging Center at Harvard. The trouble is, that knowledge is hard to come by.

It's not hard to understand the allure of stimulants, designer or otherwise. Countless baby boomers and Gen Xers have sampled cocaine and methamphetamine on a recreational basis, and will have no trouble explaining the appeal: It just feels good. In the short run, these drugs boost self-esteem, physical stamina, locomotor skills, and verbal dexterity. The original Dr. Feelgood of New York hipster fame was injecting his ultracool clientele with amphetamines. Nothing felt better than speed, if you want to put it that way.

Cathinones, like methedrine and other form of speed, are primarily dopamine-active drugs. Though they are now illegal in the U.S., they were formerly of primary interest only to pharmaceutical researchers. **The best-known cathinone sold as bath salt— mephedrone—has both dopamine and serotonin effects.** It broke big in the UK a few years ago as a "legal" party drug alternative to MDMA. Mephedrone came packaged with other chemicals under various marketing guises. And soon, as legal heat came down on the drug, designers switched to near-beer variants, and eventually began flooding the bath salt markets with other cathinone drugs whose effects were equally murky. **Users of bath salt products had been seduced, wrote Natasha Vargas-Cooper in *Spin* magazine, by the idea that they could "get high without testing dirty."**

In 2011, users of bath salt products started turning up in ERs in significant numbers. Some of them were suffering overdoses of MDMA or mephedrone, but last year a new twist on the cathinone molecular structure began to get serious traction in the states. To stay one jump ahead of the law, underground chemists began churning out large quantities of a different amphetamine variant with the tongue-twisting name of methylenedioxypyrovalerone: MDPV, for short. And what were EMTs and paramedics seeing in cases where the drug could be identified as MDPV? In a study in *Clinical Toxicology* of recent admissions involving self-reports of bath salt use, two regional poison centers reported that exposure to MDPV was becoming more common than mephedrone. And the clinical symptoms of overdose? Agitation, tachycardia, hallucinations, combative behavior, hypertension, chest pain, blurred vision—and at least one death. This synthetic cathinone was evidently capable of producing psychotic episodes requiring sedation. It all sounded eerily similar to the PCP overdoses of the 60s and 70s, when that dissociative veterinary anesthetic enjoyed a period of dubious notoriety.

The arrival of MDPV in the emergency rooms of American changed the picture considerably. Medical workers and drug enforcement officers were forced to admit that they were behind the rolling curve of drug permutations. Nobody knew what was in a given packet of bath salts or plant food, or whatever other disguise was in vogue this week. Nobody knew how much to take, or to determine how much had been taken. Doctors didn't know enough about cathinones to consistently diagnose an overdose. And what little testing was available for detecting synthetic stimulants was costly and questionable.

As 2012 began, researchers around the world were feeling pressure to find ways of discriminating between the different kinds of cathinones involved in overdoses, as a way of beginning to seriously sort out the fact from the fiction, the dangers from the overblown scare stories.

Various hopeless phrases were bandied about to describe the task of the DEA's Forensic Sciences labs—"Whack-a-Mole," "Cat-and-Mouse," and "losing battle" being among the most common. **What has them baffled and demoralized is the fact that these new chemicals under the sun were being created by underground chemists with more than casual kitchen sink skills.** And, as one undercover drug officer told *Spin* Magazine, "when you go out and seize a warehouse full of something packaged as Dragonfly, you really have no idea what it is." Nor do you know whether you can make a case against it under the Federal Analog Act, which is supposed to make all this easier by allowing cops and courts to outlaw drugs that are "substantially similar" to drugs already proscribed. Deciding questions of that nature is a matter of sophisticated biochemistry.

Dr. Michael Taffe of the Scripps Research Institute in La Jolla, CA, and pharmacology professor Annette Fleckenstein of the University of Utah have been working on these questions in the lab. Building on previous work, they had begun to conclude from their own animal studies that when it came to cathinones, there could be a big difference in effect without much evidence of a difference in chemistry.

Taffe and Fleckenstein, working separately, had produced evidence of specific behavioral differences between mephedrone and MPDV. As co-chairs of what turned out to be one of the best-attended sessions at the recent annual meeting of the College on Problems of Drug Dependence, the two scientists proceeded to expand the general understanding of a drug running rampant across three continents, and previously associated only with the chewing of Khat, a mild stimulant plant found in Africa.

Thursday, June 21, 2012

http://addiction-dirkh.blogspot.com/2012/06/low-down-on-new-highs.html

The New Highs: Are Bath Salts Addictive?

What we know and don't know about synthetic speed.

Call bath salts a new trend, if you insist. Do they cause psychosis? Are they "super-LSD?" The truth is, they are a continuation of a 70-year old trend: speed. Lately, we've been fretting about the Adderall Generation, but every population cohort has had its own confrontation with the pleasures and perils of speed: Ritalin, ice, Methedrine, crystal meth, IV meth, amphetamine, Dexedrine, Benzedrine... and so it goes. For addicts: Speed kills. Those two words were found all over posters in the Haight Ashbury district of San Francisco, a few years too late to do the residents much good.

While the matter of the addictiveness of Spice and other synthetic cannabis products remains open to question, there no longer seems to be much doubt about the stimulant drugs known collectively as bath salts. **To a greater or lesser degree, these off-the-shelf synthetic stimulants appear to be potentially addictive. And that's not good news for anyone.**

The U.S. Congress has now added 26 additional synthetic chemicals to the Controlled Substances Act, including the designer stimulants mephedrone and MDPV, at the behest of the Drug Enforcement Administration. Mephedrone and MDPV are cathinones, sold as bath salts or plant food, and chemically similar to amphetamine and ephedrine. (Methcathinone, often called MCAT, is to cathinone as methamphetamine is to amphetamine)

The research news on bath salts at the annual meeting of the College on Problems of Drug Dependence (CPDD) in Palm Springs recently was complex and confusing. **For example, the phemonenon of overheating, or hyperthermia, that plagues ravers on MDMA and sends some of them to the hospital is a function of certain temperature-sensitive effects of Ecstasy. But it is not as much of a problem with MDPV and mephedrone. The bath salts, like meth, don't seem to cause overheating as readily.**

On another front, William Fantegrossi, assistant professor in the Department of Pharmacology and Toxicology at the University of Arkansas for Medical Sciences, told the panel audience that at very high doses and very high temperatures, stimulants like Ecstasy and MDPV "can cause self-mutilation in animals." Fantegrossi's statement was the closest anybody has come to providing a possible scientific basis for popular press accounts linking bath salts to flesh-eating frenzies by psychotic users. But this remains speculative.

The symposium on bath salts at the CPDD played to a packed conference hall, a sure sign that professional scientists who study addiction for a living were interested in the subject. The panel was titled "A Stimulating Soak in 'Bath Salts': Investigating Cathinone Derivative Drugs," and was co-chaired by Dr. Michael Taffe of the Scripps Research Institute in La Jolla, CA, and pharmacology professor Dr. Annette Fleckenstein of the University of Utah.

Fantegrossi characterized the overall problem of designer stimulants as "dirty pharmacology" on both sides, pointing to the desperate efforts underway by government-funded scientists to "throw antagonists [blocking drugs] at these things."

Alexander Shulgin, the grandfather of the modern psychedelic movement, popularized MDMA and hundreds of variants in his backyard laboratory in the Bay Area over the years. Shulgin, better than anyone, knew that legitimate research and dirty recreational chemistry are only a molecule away. In their book *Pihkal: A Chemical Love Story,* Alexander Shulgin and his wife Ana recall that cartoonist Gary Trudeau captured the truth of the situation as far back as 1985, when the MDMA story became front-page news:

Way back in mid-1985, the cartoonist-author of Doonesbury, Gary Trudeau, did a two-week feature on it, playing it humorous, and almost (but not quite) straight, in a hilarious sequence of twelve strips. On August 19, 1985 he had Duke, president of Baby Doc College, introduce the drug design team from USC in the form of two brilliant twins, Drs. Albie and Bunny Gorp. They vividly demonstrated to the enthusiastic conference that their new drug "Intensity" was simply MDMA with one of the two oxygens removed. "Voila," said one of them, with a molecular model in his hands, "Legal as sea salt."

Jeffrey Moran of the Arkansas Department of Health noted that despite the cat-and-mouse game continuously played between illegal drug designers and the law, government bans on mephedrone and MDPV, the two most common forms of designer stimulant, cause only temporary downturns in supply. They are no longer as legal as sea salt, but it doesn't seem to matter. There are always new ones in the pipeline. **Moran told the audience that at least 48 different compounds had been identified in more than 200 distinct bath salt-style products in his state alone.** Sorting out the specific chemistry involves specialized assays designed to detect a bewildering array of molecules: methylone, mephedrone, paphyrone, butylone, 4-MEC, alpha-PVP, and a host of others, some old, some new, some reimagined by underground chemists.

Terry Boos of the U.S. Drug Enforcement Agency explained that most designer stimulants currently in play are not manufactured stateside. **Most originate in Asia and arrive through various ports of call, where they are repackaged for sale in the U.S. Purity of the cathinone ranges from 30 to 95 per cent, Boos said.**

Annette Fleckenstein of the University of Utah emphasized that scientists shouldn't be fooled by overall structural similarities among such drugs as meth, mephedrone, MDMA, and MDPV. In a 2011 study published with her colleagues at the University of Utah, Fleckenstein lamented that mephedrone's recent emergence on the drug scene had exposed the fact that "there are no formal pharmacodynamic or pharmacokinetic studies of mephedrone."

But she has managed to show that methamphetamine causes lasting decreases in serotonin functions, as well as the better-known dopamine alterations, and that MDMA and mephedrone are intimately involved in the accumulation of serotonin in the brain's nucleus accumbens, where addictive drugs produce many of their rewarding effects. **"Rats will self-administer mephedrone," said Fleckenstein—always a troubling clue that the drug in question may have addictive properties**. Since the high in humans only lasts for three to six hours, there is a tendency to reinforce the behavior through repeated dosings.

Other behavioral clues have been teased out of rat studies. The Taffe Laboratory at Scripps Research Institute has focused on the cognitive, thermoregulatory, and potentially addictive effects of the cathinones. Rats will self-administer mephedrone, MDPV, and of course methamphetamine. However, Dr. Taffe told the audience that MDMA does not produce these classic locomotor stimulant effects at low doses and that it is "more difficult to get them to self-administer" Ecstasy. Nonetheless, Taffe told me he believes that MDMA is, in fact, potentially addictive. **"Our data suggest that MDPV is highly reinforcing," Taffe said in an email exchange after the conference, "and at least as readily self-administered** as methamphetamine, at approximately the same per-infusion doses. But it is a very complicated story."

Scripps researchers have carried the investigation forward with a new study in the journal *Drug and Alcohol Dependence*. Pai-Kai Huang and coworkers studied the differing effects of designer stimulants on voluntary wheel-running activity in rats, adding additional evidence to the basic behavioral split among club drugs of the moment. Taffe, one of the study's co-authors, said the researchers had predicted that the two drugs with the strongest serotonin activity—MDMA and the mephedrone variants—would *decrease* wheel running activity in the rats. Methedrine and MDPV, they predicted, would *increase* activity.

And that's how it turned out. What that means for human users is still not entirely clear. **But MDPV in particular, it now seems evident, has some rather direct and disturbing affinities with crystal meth and cocaine.** And the vagaries of the market have led to sharp increases in the percentage of MDPV found in bath salt products in the last two years. Are we seeing the wholesale replacement of MDMA by a more directly addictive, methedrine-like drug? Will we see a rise in psychotic symptoms, and increased visits to the ER, as MDPV becomes more common in bath salts? Ecstasy has been implicated in the death of users as well, but will the surge in cathinone drugs mean there will be additional deaths?

And remember: Researchers are able to distinguish between rats under the influence of either MDMA- or MDPV-based wheel activity—but the research suggests that under blinded conditions, human users aren't very good at guessing which of those two drugs they're on. Furthermore, we don't have the data to say whether users can tell mephedrone from MDPV in a blind test. And even wheel-running rats don't give away whether they're running on MDMA or mephedrone. These categorical distinctions are all-important, but still in relative infancy as far as street use is concerned.

The Scripps scientists concluded that their study "underlines the error of assuming all novel cathinone derivative stimulants that become popular with recreational users will share neuropharmacological or biobehavioral properties." Some of the combinations produce a "unique constellation of desired effects."

But by 2011, the U.S. media had conflated mephedrone with MDPV and half a dozen other substances, all with differing effects on users. For public health officials, it was a nightmare.

"We know that MDMA users follow the science," Taffe said, at the close of the bath salts panel. "So information we make available can have a direct effect on public health for those people." But for bath salt users, the picture is not as clear. Consider, once again, Arkansas' finding of 30 or 40 different cathinone derivatives, part of a set of 250 distinct chemicals identified in different combinations of bath salt products. "Slight modifications can change the toxicities," Taffe said. "Abuse liabilities differ between MDMA and different cathinones. They all confer different health risks."

One of the primary drivers of bath salt usage appears to be the desire to finesse drug-testing programs. And if drug-testing programs are pushing people in the direction of more dangerous, unfamiliar, and addictive substances, then perhaps drug testing is part of the problem rather than the solution.

In the short run, emergency treatment of patients with OD symptoms they attribute to bath salts will remain the same, whether the cathinone in question is mephedrone, MDPV, or some other variant. General emergency-department procedures for stimulant intoxication are standardized. People can suffer cardiac arrest from either MDMA or meth. And people can run very high temperatures with overdoses of any of these stimulants.

Are users listening? Do they believe any of the health warnings this time out, or have there been too many over the years, always strident and hysterical and overinflated?

Tuesday, June 26, 2012

http://addiction-dirkh.blogspot.com/2012/06/new-highs-are-bath-salts-addictive.html

Huang PK, Aarde SM, Angrish D, Houseknecht KL, Dickerson TJ, & Taffe MA. Contrasting effects of d-methamphetamine, 3,4-methylenedioxymethamphetamine, 3,4-methylenedioxypyrovalerone, and 4-methylmethcathinone on wheel activity in rats. Drug and alcohol dependence. 2012. PMID: 22664136

Khat to the Chase

Of mephedrone, bath salts, and impaired driving.

Automobile accidents are the ninth leading cause of death worlwide, according to the World Health Organization (WHO). More than a million people are killed on roads annually, and that number could rise to 2.5 million by 2020. WHO estimates that traffic accidents cost developing countries an astonishing 1-2 % of their gross domestic product (GDP).

For years now, police and public health officials have puzzled over the alarming number of traffic accidents in East Africa. In terms of sheer numbers, Asian countries have the highest total traffic fatalities, according to figures compiled by the Global Road Safety Partnership (GRSP), a consortium including the World Bank, the Red Cross and other aid agencies. That is not surprising, since these nations contain the majority of the world's drivers.

However, beyond the picture of traffic fatalities in terms of sheer numbers, or on a per population basis, there is another revealing measure—traffic deaths per motor vehicle. And when the GRSP measured nations by that yardstick, the four worst countries in the world for traffic deaths—judging by the number of fatalities per 10,000 licensed vehicles—were Ethiopia, Tanzania, Lesotho, and Kenya—all East African nations.

Moreover, these are all African countries in which the use of khat–an amphetamine-like plant drug that is the natural precursor of the designer drug known as mephedrone—is legal and common. The major khat-using countries in Africa are commonly listed as: Somalia, Kenya, Yemen, Ethiopa, Tanzania, Lesotho. Note the overlap. **Khat, as one online article put it, is "the legal high of east Africa."**

On the tiny island nation of Mauritius, just off the southeast African coast, Touria Prayag writes at allAfrica.com that drivers "zoom past you, zigzag on the roads, nervously changing to the left lane to swiftly veer back on your side without any warning.... brazenly flouting the Highway Code in every imaginable dangerous manner.... And the carnage continues...."

In Ethiopia, annual road crash fatalities account for 114 deaths per 10,000 vehicles, compared to one death per 10,000 vehicles in Great Britain, and an average of 60 deaths per 10,000 vehicles across 39 sub-Saharan African countries. A report in the *Bulletin of the World Health Organization* notes that Ethiopian truck drivers "are regarded as so dangerous that their trucks are commonly referred to across Ethiopia as 'al Qaeda.'" Anecdotally, Ethiopians told WHO officials that khat "increased driver confidence and vehicle speed while also making drivers irritable and impairing concentration," and that high levels of khat could lead to hallucinations.

A Kenya forum on TripAdvisor asks: Are matatus [local taxis piloted by khat-chewing Kenyans] safe?"

Since khat is legally available in most of East Africa, and comprises a significant part of the social fabric of local cultures, the use of khat is similar to the use of alcohol in higher-income nations. But does khat present the same threat of driving impairment as alcohol? Bolivia is now arguing its right to allow citizens to chew coca leaves in the traditional manner. Is it safe to drive and chew coca leaves? In all of these cases, the challenge is to determine what constitutes a "safe" dose of the drug; a dose that does not endanger people on or near the highway. There is not enough research on khat to answer that question. Nor is there a way to administer roadside tests for khat. The best evidence, African police officers say, is green teeth.

The active ingredients in khat—cathine and cathinone—are similar in structure to amphetamines, and chemically similar to the ingredients used in the manufacture of mephedrone powder. Mephedrone is sold as 4-MMC, Meow Meow, M-Cat, and other nicknames. Cathine and cathinone ramp up dopamine, serotonin and noradrenaline levels in a manner very similar to amphetamine, with many of the same positive effects (mild euphoria, reduced hunger, increased energy) and the same negative effects (depression, fatigue, lack of appetite, drug craving). **It is thought that chronic use of khat results in dopamine D2 depletion in areas of the brain involved in goal-directed action.**

The current fervor over mephedrone being disguised as bath salts or plant food for black market sales purposes in the U.S and U.K. demonstrates that this question is not academic for developed western nations. Sold as Ivory Wave, or Bliss, or White Lightning, mephedrone and other products containing cathinone are increasingly available across the U.S. states. **In 2008, police seized 600 pounds of fresh khat—in Fargo, North Dakota.**

A recent paper published in *Frontiers in Psychology*, authored by a group of Dutch and Spanish psychologists, appears to show that khat users exhibit a specific cognitive deficit: **On stop-signal tasks, stop signal reaction time (SSRT) was significantly slower for the khat users.** Such tests typically involve rapidly pressing a green "go" button upon seeing an arrow in certain positions, or abruptly aborting the response when the arrow turns red. The test measures "individual ability to stop a planned or ongoing motor response in a voluntary fashion." For example, someone with

Parkinson's disease would score at the very high end of the SSRT scale.

The study itself involved 20 regular khat users recruited from the immigrant populations of Leiden and The Hague, and matched against 20 khat-free controls. All of the khat users met four or more of the 7 DSM-IV criteria for addiction, and did not consume alcohol the night before the test. The investigators speculate that this reduced level of inhibitory control "may even be involved in the emergence of addiction: the more a drug is used, the less able users are to prevent themselves from using it."

The parallels to traffic signals and stop signs are obvious, and apt. The authors state that the findings of their study are "rather worrying because, first, many real-life situations require active inhibition of prepotent actions, as in the case of traffic lights turning red, or of criminal actions." **The obvious conclusion is that the chronic chewing of khat leaves "may indeed lead to a marked deterioration of cognitive functions (as inhibitory control) implicated in driving behavior."** Studies by NIDA director Nora Volkow and others have show that cocaine users suffer similar reductions in dopamine D2 receptors and "need significantly more time to inhibit responses to stop signals than non-users." In general, stimulant drugs taken regularly at high doses appear to disrupt response inhibition due to alterations in dopamine functioning. (Although some studies have shown a facilitation of inhibitory control at lower doses).

The usual caveats apply: It is impossible to rule out pre-existing propensities for impulsivity, disinhibition, and the like. Some health researchers do not agree that the case for driving impairment on khat has yet been made. **In the *Bulletin of the World Health Organization*, Anita Feigin of the Centre for Population Health in Australia writes that, so far, much of the information is anecdotal, "and, as yet, there is no clear evidence**

of a causal relationship between the use of khat and traffic accidents." African taxi drivers who immigrate to Australia use khat "to stay awake and alert." However, Feigin notes that the use of khat has deeply divided the members of east African migrant communities.

It is an interesting conundrum. The developed West has its entrenched tradition of alcohol as a legal high, despite its side-effects, which frequently result in mayhem on the highways. On the other hand, the drinking nations must now contend with demands from other cultures for the decriminalization of khat and coca leaf, which, along with coffee and tea, make up a category we might call the "soft" stimulants.

Because of the connection with mephedrone and other amphetamine-like designer drugs, these questions will not be going away until more research provides some solid answers. Such research may not be long in coming: The NIH-funded Khat Research Program (KRP) at the University of Minnesota, for example, brings American researchers together with a broad group of scientists from Yemenese and German universities to study the effects of a common plant drug most Americans have never heard of—but a drug they may be dealing with in synthetic form sooner rather than later.

Wednesday, January 26, 2011

http://addiction-dirkh.blogspot.com/2011/01/khat-to-chase.html

Colzato, L., Ruiz, M., van den Wildenberg, W., Bajo, M., & Hommel, B.. Long-Term Effects of Chronic Khat Use: Impaired Inhibitory Control *Frontiers in Psychology.* 2011. DOI: 10.3389/fpsyg.2010.00219

"Bath Salts" and Ecstasy Implicated in Kidney Injuries

"A potentially life-threatening situation."

In March of 2012, state officials became alarmed by a cluster of puzzling health problems that had suddenly popped up in Casper, Wyoming, population 55,000. Three young people had been hospitalized with kidney injuries, and dozens of others were allegedly suffering from vomiting and back pain after smoking or snorting an herbal product sold as "blueberry spice." The *Poison Review* reported that the outbreak was presently under investigation by state medical officials. "At this point we are viewing use of this drug as a potentially life-threatening situation," said Tracy Murphy, Wyoming state epidemiologist.

It is beginning to look like acute kidney injury from the newer synthetic drugs may be a genuine threat. And if that wasn't bad enough, continuing research has implicated MDMA, better known as Ecstasy, as another potential source of kidney damage. Recreational druggies, forewarned is forearmed.

Bath salts first. In the Wyoming case, while the drug in question may have been one of the synthetic marijuana products marketed as Spice, it's entirely possible that the drug in question was actually one or more of the new synthetic stimulants called bath salts. (Quality control and truth in packaging are not part of this industry). The *American Journal of Kidney Diseases* recently published a report titled "Recurrent Acute Kidney Injury Following Bath Salts Intoxication." It features a case history that Yale researchers believe to be "the first report of recurrent acute kidney injury associated with repeated bath salts intoxication." The most common causes for emergency room admissions due to bath salts—primarily the drugs MDPV and mephedrone—are agitation, hallucinations, and tachycardia, the authors report. But the case report of a 26-year old man showed recurrent kidney injury after using bath salts. The authors speculate that the damage resulted from "severe renal vasospasm induced by these vasoactive substances." (A vasoactive substance can constrict or dilate blood vessels.)

A possible secondary mechanism of action for kidney damage among bath salt users is rhabdomyolysis— a breakdown of muscle fibers that releases muscle fiber contents into the bloodstream, causing severe kidney damage. Heavy alcohol and drug use, especially cocaine, are also known risk factors for this condition. The complicating factor here is that rhabdomyolysis has also been described in cases of MDMA intoxication, and here we arrive at the second part of the story.

In 2008, the *Clinical Journal of the American Society of Nephrology* published "The Agony of Ecstasy: MDMA and the Kidney." In this study, Garland A. Campbell and Mitchell H. Rosner of the University of Virginia Department of Medicine found that "Ecstasy has been associated with acute kidney injury that is most commonly secondary to nontraumatic rhabdomyolysis but also has been reported in the setting of drug-induced liver failure and drug-induced vasculitis."

Chemically, MDMA is another amphetamine spinoff, like mephedrone and other bath salts. Many people take this club drug regularly without apparent harm, whereas others seem to be acutely sensitive and can experience serious toxicity, possibly due to genetic variance in the breakdown enzyme CYP2D6. The authors trace the first case report of acute kidney injury due to Ecstasy back to 1992, but "because most of these data are accrued from case reports, the absolute incidence of this complication cannot be determined."

Campbell and Rosner believe that nontraumatic rhabdomyolysis is a likely culprit in many cases, and speculate that the condition is "greatly compounded by the ambient temperature, which in crowded rave parties is usually elevated." If a physician suspects rhabdomyolysis in an Ecstasy user, "aggressive cooling measures should be undertaken to lower the patient's core temperature to levels that will lessen further muscle and end-organ injury." This complication can have far-reaching effects: The authors note the case history of "transplant graft loss of both kidneys obtained from a donor with a history of recent Ecstasy use."

In addition, there may be undocumented risks to the liver as well. An earlier study by Andreu and others claims that "up to 31% of all drug toxicity-related acute hepatic failure is due to MDMA... Patients with severe acute hepatic failure secondary to ecstasy use often survive with supportive care and have successfully undergone liver transplantation."

But the picture is far from clear: "Unfortunately, no case reports of acute kidney injury secondary to Ecstasy have had renal biopsies performed to allow for further elucidation..." And attributing firm causation is difficult, due to the fact that MDMA users often use other drugs in combination, some of which, like cocaine, can cause kidney problem all by themselves.

A study by Harold Kalant of the University of Toronto's Addiction Research Foundation, published in the *Canadian Medical Association Journal*, proposed that **"dantrolene, which is a drug used to stop the intense muscle contractures in malignant hyperthermia, should also be useful in the hyperthermic**

type of MDMA toxicity. Numerous cases have now been treated in this way, some with rapid and dramatic results even when the clinical picture suggested the likelihood of a fatal outcome."

Sunday, March 18, 2012

http://addiction-dirkh.blogspot.com/2012/03/bath-salts-and-ecstasy-implicated-in.html

Adebamiro, A., and Perazella, M. Recurrent Acute Kidney Injury Following Bath Salts Intoxication *American Journal of Kidney Diseases,* *59* (2), 273-275. 2012. DOI: 10.1053/j.ajkd.2011.10.012

The Triumph of Synthetics

Designer stimulants surpass heroin and cocaine.

A troubling 2011 report by the United Nations Office on Drugs and Crime (UNODC) shows that amphetamine-type stimulants (ATS) have, for the first time, become more popular around the world than heroin and cocaine. Marijuana remains the most popular illegal drug in the world, and the use of amphetamines has fallen sharply in the U.S., but the world trend represents the worldwide triumph of synthetic drug design over the plant-based "hard drugs" of the past.

The 2011 Global ATS Assessment estimates that in 2009, some 14 to 57 million people aged 15-64 took an amphetamine-type substance during the year. The category includes methamphetamine, synthetic stimulants known as bath salts, and Ecstasy. For ecstasy, which is grouped with the ATS family because of its speed-like qualities, "global annual prevalence" stood at only 11-28 million past-year users in 2009, basically unchanged. Not so for the use of the new synthetic methamphetamines—compounds such as mephedrone, 4-methylmethcathinone (4-MMC) and MDPV, which first took off in the UK, Canada, and New Zealand. In fact, bath salts in the form of mephedrone are competing with ecstasy as the club drug of the moment. (Ecstasy seizures are currently at a 5-year high in the United States, so the window for alternatives is currently wide open.) **Meanwhile, recorded worldwide use of heroin, cocaine, and marijuana remained essentially steady from 2005 to 2009.**

So what's behind the global surge in production of amphetamine-type drugs? What advantages do these stimulants hold over time-tested drugs like heroin and coke? And why is it happening now?

The seismic changes in worldwide drug production begin with geography. Amphetamine-type stimulants are spreading to new regions, and are now being manufactured in places previously off the radar—Iran, Malaysia, and West Africa, for starters. The UNODC report notes that synthetic stimulants "offer criminals a new entry into unexploited and fresh markets." The locus of activity is no longer the opium fields of Afghanistan, or the coca plantations of Columbia. **In absolute numbers, the report claims, "most ATS users live in Southeast Asia, the most populous sub-region the world."**

The growing number of methamphetamine pills seized in Southeast Asia is staggering: "The 93.3 million methamphetamine pills seized in 2009 in China, Lao People's Democratic Republic, Myanmar and Thailand represent a three-fold increase in comparison with 2008 figures," the UN report alleges. "In 2010, total seizures surpassed 133 million pills." Not since the Japanese amphetamine scourge of the post-World War II years has East Asia seen anything like this.

The UN report singles out two new countries—Lao People's Democratic Republic, and Malaysia—as nations reporting, for the first time, "the injecting use of crystalline methamphetamine in 2008 and 2009." And a massive increase in production has been documented in northern Burma. *Voice of America News* **reports that amphetamine-type drug seizures in Burma went from one million pills in 2008 to a mind-blowing 23 million pills a year later.**

A regional representative for the UNODC in East Asia said that the seizures "reflect a dramatic increase in production in the Shan State" in Northern Burma. The production of methamphetamine is a primary source of income for the Shan, whose territory is near the borders of China and Thailand. "What we are worried about," said the UNODC rep, "is the nexus of drugs, of weapons, of money that is moving around that region at a time when elections are pending and the political situation is quite fragile." At the same time, Burma remains a major supplier of opiates, though competition with Afghanistan may have helped encourage the production of illegal stimulants. UNODC Executive Director Yury Fedotove explained that the market for synthetic stimulants "has evolved from a cottage-type industry typified by small-scale manufacturing operations to more of a cocaine or heroin-type market with a higher level of integration and organized crime groups involved throughout the production and supply chain."

Amphetamines, in all their synthetic forms, have several production advantages over plant-based addictive drugs like heroin and cocaine. In recent years, the U.S. and other countries have cracked down on amphetamine precursor drugs like ephedrine and pseudoephedrine. Once these tried and true compounds for amphetamine manufacture—found in cold and allergy medications—were registered and controlled, traffickers made the switch to different chemical approaches. **New building blocks like phelylacetic acid and l-phenylacetylcarbinol (l-PAC) have been found in labs from Canada to Mexico.** Growers of opium and coca have no such alternatives available to them. Pharmacologist David Kroll, Professor and Chair of Pharmaceutical Science at North Carolina Central University in Durham, who has been following the new synthetic drug products on his blog, Terra Sigillata, said that some of the latest precursors have a problematic history. "Phenylacetate and phelylacetic acid have been investigated in clinical trials for cancer and in the treatment of sickle cell disease," said Dr. Kroll. "But they didn't fare well in large clinical trails because they required such high doses, and patients had side effects."

While this is definitely not a reliable class of compounds from which to fashion new recreational stimulants, Dr. Kroll noted that rendering synthetic drugs illegal can sometimes play havoc with efforts to develop the same drugs for therapeutic purposes. **"If these precursors become more strictly regulated, there might be an untoward effect on the prices of other drugs" that use the same compound as a building block, he said.**

Drug lab seizures in Jordan, Syria, and the United Arab Emirates have also reached new highs—particularly the clandestine manufacture of a form of amphetamine called phenethylline, marketed under the brand name Captagon. Very little in the way of equipment or startup capital is required, which facilitates new players in this market. Captagon, said Dr. Kroll, "makes pretty good sense. The body can metabolize it to amphetamine itself—it's an amphetamine pro-drug. The other metabolite of the drug is theophylline, the old asthma drug that also acts as a mild stimulant. But it's potentially as dangerous as amphetamine, depending on how efficient one's metabolism is." This is, of course, a huge problem: **One bath salts user might have an acceptable drug experience, while another might find that a few whiffs of the same synthetic stimulant will land him or her in the emergency room, with a dangerously elevated heart rate or other complications.**

What drug designers, drug manufacturers, and drug suppliers have come to realize is that methamphetamine and other ATS drugs appear to fill the lifestyle void left by the uncertain supply and pricing situation associated with cocaine. Everywhere they land, synthetic stimulants—from biker crank to mephedrone—wreak instant havoc. They simply are not predictable compounds. One bath salts user compared the experience to "a shot of methamphetamine with a PCP chaser." From any kind of rational sociocultural point of view, these are not safe drugs. And it hardly needs repeating that they are highly addictive for many people. The legalization of amphetamine is not a cause likely to gain much momentum any time soon.

Even though the United States has a long history of dealing with amphetamine, this is manifestly not true of every country in the world. And now these untapped markets are fair game for cheaper, longer lasting amphetamine-type stimulants, which "seem to appeal to the needs of today's societies and have become part of what is perceived to be a modern and dynamic lifestyle," according to the UNODC report.

We don't know with complete certainty that the drug data coming out of several key areas—Southeast Asia, Africa, and the Middle East in particular—is accurate. Authorities have captured and dismantled ATS labs in Central and South America as well. In all likelihood, drug production and use in all these regions is underreported. The UNODC document laments that "household and other surveys are lacking or are outdated in some countries in several of the most affected regions." This is a particular problem in China and India, where no serious national survey of amphetamine-type stimulants has ever been undertaken.

We have a long way to go before we know the outcome of the current craze for synthetic stimulants. The historical wreckage caused by injected methedrine in the 60s and 70s, and smokable ice in the 90s and the aughts, is a grisly matter of public record. Now we are confronted with a baffling cornucopia of designer concoctions whose track record for safe recreation is, thus far, not so good. Amphetamine drugs have sent thousands to their deaths, and countless others to the emergency rooms. And now this deadly deck of stimulants has many more cards in it than it did just a few years ago. Pick a card, any card. First one's free.

Tuesday, November 29, 2011

http://addiction-dirkh.blogspot.com/2011/11/triumph-of-synthetics.html

3) Treatment

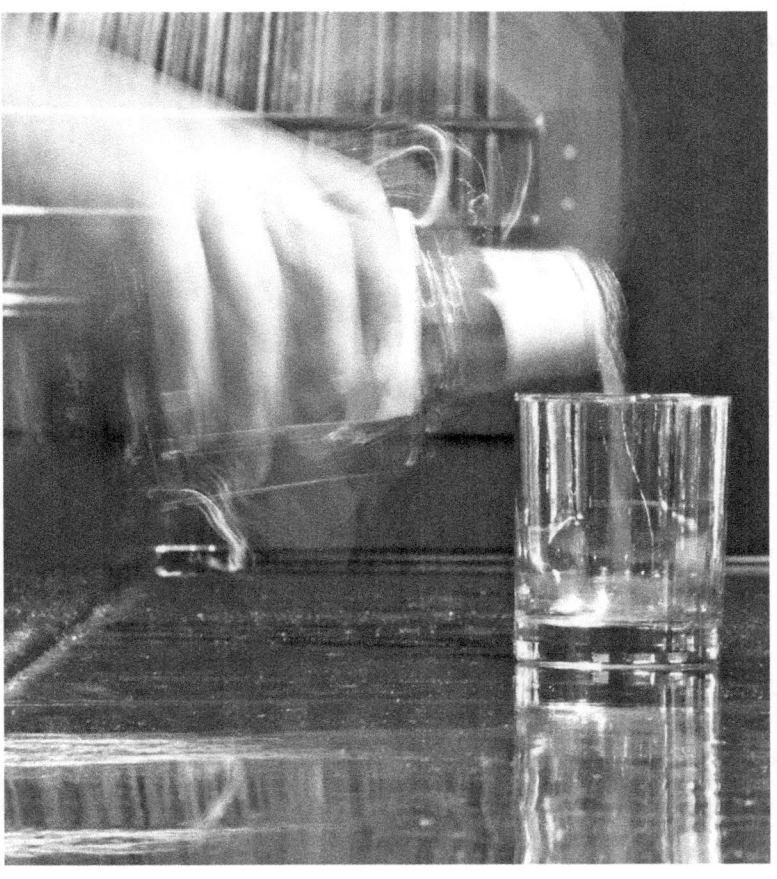

(Photo by Peter Hanson)

The Three-Headed Dragon

A symbol of need.

Getting off drugs, or learning to stop drinking, is very often easier than staying off them. As Mark Twain remarked about tobacco, quitting was easy—he'd done it dozens of times. Relapse, the biological imperative, will have its way with most of those abstaining for the first time. Addiction is a psychological disorder with strongly cued behavioral components, whatever its dimensions as a biochemically-based disease.

The three-headed dragon is a metaphor first popularized by alternative therapists at the Haight Ashbury Free Medical Clinic in San Francisco. The first head of the dragon is physical. Addiction is a chronic illness requiring a lifetime of attention. The second head is psychological. Addiction is a disorder with mental, emotional, and behavioral components. And the third head of the dragon is spiritual. Addiction is an existential state, experienced in isolation from others.

Addicts speak of "chasing the dragon" in an effort to catch the high that they used to achieve so easily. It is also drug slang for the use of small metal pipes to catch and inhale the wisps of smoke from a pile of burning opium, crack, or speed. **We can picture the dragon chasing his own tail, snapping at it with all three hungry mouths, in an endless escalation of tolerance and need.**

"Because of the unique reaction that the genetically addiction-prone individual experiences to his drug of choice, he or she programs his or her belief system with the deep conviction that the substance is 'good,'" writes Richard Seymour. "This is where self-help becomes intrinsic to recovery. Unless one deals with the third head, unless one changes the belief system and effects a turning-about in the deepest seat of consciousness, there is no recovery." The "X" factor in recovery, for many people, turns out to be a form of inner self-awareness; something that includes the attributes of will power and determination yet transcends them through a form of surrender.

And speaking of changing one's belief system, experience has shown that it is a spectacularly bad idea to sit around and do nothing but stare at the wall during the early phase of recovery. Psychologist Mihaly Csikszentmihalyi argues, in *The Evolving Self*, that when attention wanders, and goal-directed action wanes, the majority of thoughts that come to mind tend to be depressive or sad. (This does not necessarily apply to formal methods of meditation, which cannot be described as states marked by wandering attention.) The reason that the mind turns to negative thoughts under such conditions, he writes, is that such pessimism may be evolutionarily adaptive. "The mind turns to negative possibilities as a compass needle turns to the magnetic pole, because this is the best way, on the average, to anticipate dangerous situations." In the case of recovering addicts, this anticipation of dangerous situations is known as craving. The next step is often drug-seeking behavior, followed by relapse.

For a highly motivated addict with a stable social life, a safe and effective medication to combat craving might be all that is needed. For many others, however, attention to the other two heads of the dragon is going to be necessary. An addict's ability to experience pleasure in the normal way has been biochemically impaired. It takes time for the addict's disordered pleasure system to begin returning to normal, just as it takes time for the physical damage of cigarette smoking to partially repair itself.

Alternative therapists are fond of referring to recovery as a process, with an emphasis on the importance of time. Medication of any disease, even if successful, does not treat the continuing need for healing. It is now well understood that mood and outlook can have an effect on healing. Positive emotional states can be beneficial to the maintenance of good health. Thoughtful physicians make the distinction between a disease and an illness. A disease is a chemically identifiable pathological process. An illness, by contrast, is the disease and all that surrounds it—the sociological environment, and the individual psychology of the patient who experiences the disease.

Sunday, January 31, 2010

http://addiction-dirkh.blogspot.com/2010/01/three-headed-dragon.html

From The Chemical Carousel By Dirk Hanson, pp. 311-313. © Dirk Hanson, 2008.

Needle Exchange in America

AIDS/harm reduction activists press Obama.

First, the good news: After 20 years, the U.S. Congress has voted to remove the funding ban on syringe exchange programs designed to combat AIDS and to bring hard drug users within the orbit of the medical health community.

Now, the bad news: Conservative legislators have managed to insert a provision in the bill prohibiting needle exchange centers within 1,000 feet of schools, day care centers, colleges, playgrounds, youth centers, swimming pools—and just about any other institution you care to come up with. In short, the legislation would make it virtually impossible to operate a viable needle exchange program, even if sufficient levels of federal funding can be obtained. As one harm reduction activist put it in the *Seattle Stranger*: **The only place you could put a federally-funded needle exchange program in the entire city of Chicago... is O'Hare Airport?** Gee, it's almost like Democrats aren't really serious about allowing funding live-saving needle programs at all."

Clearly, needle exchange activists are still waiting for an unambiguous sign from the White House that Obama plans to uphold his campaign promises in this regard. **Obama's go-slow policy on needle exchange has frustrated AIDS activists in particular.**

Physicians for Human Rights, a group that supports clean syringe exchange programs, made October 14, 2009 a National

Call-in Day, noting on its web site that "Senators need to hear from President Obama that his Administration supports syringe exchange. Now is the time to urge President Obama to fulfill his campaign promise to end the ban and to urge the Senate to act."

Earlier this year, I wrote: "Obama's agenda, as spelled out at Whitehouse.gov, calls for rescinding the ban in an effort to save lives by reducing the transmission of HIV/AIDS. 'The President,' according to the agenda, 'supports lifting the federal ban on needle exchange, which could dramatically reduce rates of infection among drug users.'"

Syringe exchange programs, Physicians for Human Rights declares, "do more than provide clean syringes and properly dispose of used ones; they link people into the health care system and drug treatment programs that save lives."

In short, says the group, "the presence of syringe exchange programs in communities does not increase rates of drug use, nor does it lead to a rise in crime. What it does do: decrease transmission of HIV, Hepatitis C and other diseases."

Moreover, during his confirmation hearings drug czar Gil Kerlikowske said that "a number of studies conducted in the US have shown needle exchange programs do not increase drug use."

It's a confusing picture in the field: Needle exchange programs exist, in San Francisco, Toronto, New York and other major metropolitan areas, because county and other local and regional officials have authorized it, even when funding was precarious. Alongside these programs, a plethora of illegal needle exchange operations is also in place. The *Drug War Chronicle* quoted the Western director of the Harm Reduction Coalition: **"We need to get legislation authorizing syringe exchanges on a statewide level.... Requiring local authorization means we have to deal with 54 jurisdictions instead of just one."**

Back in May, Maia Szalavitz reported in *Time* that the president was planning to move deliberately as part of a broader HIV/AIDS strategy, even though groups from the World Health Organization (WHO) to the American Medical Association have gone on record with the view that giving clean needles to drug addicts is a successful strategy to reduce the spread of HIV disease. Studies by Don Des Jarlais of Beth Israel Hospital in New York suggest that infection rates in New York's drug addict population may have dropped more than 75 % over the last few years as clean needle programs became increasingly available.

In a report last month by the Drug Reform Coordination Effort (DRCNet), a spokesperson for the AIDS Action group was determined to remain positive. **"I have a pretty good feeling about this," he said. "I'm hopeful this is the year."**

Friday, November 6, 2009

http://addiction-dirkh.blogspot.com/2009/11/needle-exchange-in-america.html

Army Doctor Sees Victory, and a Dangerous Drug Bites the Dust Almost

An interview with the man who blew the whistle on the neurotoxic malaria drug in the U.S. Army's kit bag.

A dangerous malaria drug invented by the Army and commonly used by soldiers and civilians alike causes everything from episodes of psychotic violence to nightmares more real than reality, and is finally being withdrawn as the first-line treatment for troops in malarial zones.

Lariam, known medically as mefloquine, has also been a licensed treatment for civilians abroad for more than 25 years. Yet it has only been in the recent past that common knowledge of Lariam's dangers has surfaced publically.

The development of Lariam was a prime example of military-industrial cooperation. Discovered at the Walter Reed Army Institute of Research during the Vietnam war, initially tested on prisoners at the Joliet Correctional Center in Illinois, and marketed worldwide by Hoffmann-La Roche, mefloquine was an urgent response to high malaria rates in U.S. combat troops overseas. Unfortunately, such close cooperation also led to a lack of adequate clinical testing—the practice that underpins the notion of drug safety. Ashley M. Croft

185

of the Royal Army Medical Corps in Britain has written that in the case of Lariam, "the first randomized controlled trial of the drug in a mixed population of general travellers was not reported until 2001." Croft believes the FDA was influenced by "the powerful military-industrial-governmental lobby into over-hasty decisions."

In addition, "travel medicine experts in most countries were slow to recognize the danger signals associated with Lariam.... As late as 2005 a reviewer in the *New England Journal of Medicine*, also an employee of the US military for over 20 years, continued to maintain... that Lariam was a 'well tolerated' drug," according to Croft. The victims of all this pharmacological hoodoo, Croft maintains, "have been those many business travellers, embassy staff, tourists, aid workers, missionaries, soldiers and others who were well at the start of their journeys into malaria-endemic areas..."

Largely due to the efforts of Dr. Remington Nevin, a medical epidemiologist and a physician in the U.S. Army, who went public about Lariam's potential for causing psychological illness, military officials announced in December that the Army was done with Lariam as a first-line malaria preventative except for "special circumstances." In the past, such special circumstances have allegedly included its use as an interrogation drug at Guantanamo.

As far back as 2004, an alarming number of suicides among troops in Iraq prompted calls for an investigation of Lariam. "The military is ignoring this drug's known side effects," Steve Robinson of the National Gulf War Resource Center told *UPI*. In October of 2004, Sen. Dianne Feinstein (D-Calif) urged then-Secretary of Defense Donald Rumsfeld to investigate the drug: "Given the mounting concerns about Lariam as expressed by civilians, service members and medical experts about its known serious side effects, I strongly urge you to reassess," she wrote to Rumsfeld. Meanwhile, Mark Benjamin and Dan Olmsted of *UPI* were reporting that "mounting evidence suggests Lariam has triggered mental problems so severe that in a small percentage of users it has led to suicide. *UPI* also reported that soldiers involved in a string of murder-suicides at Fort Bragg, N.C., in the summer of 2002 after returning from Afghanistan had taken the drug."

Almost ten years later, Sen. Feinstein wrote another letter, this one to Secretary of Defense Leon Panetta, complaining that a 2009 policy limiting the use of mefloquine among U.S. troops was not being followed. **Although parent company Roche discontinued Lariam in the U.S., generic versions remain available, and the company continues to sell Lariam in other countries.** "My office has been contacted recently by servicemembers who were prescribed mefloquine when one of the other medications would have been appropriate and were not given the FDA information card. These servicemembers are now suffering from preventable neurological side effects," including balance problems, vertigo, and psychotic behavior, she wrote.

In addition, as a military medical instructor told Addiction Inbox: "Some service members might 'double up' on their weekly dose, or increase the frequency of dosing, intentionally for recreational purposes. There is no evidence that the military educates service members to avoid this temptation or that it is unsafe. Users might even justify it by believing it could enhance the drug's anti-malarial activity. In the military, it is frequently a tenet of our culture that 'if one is good, two is better.'"

In November, military officials overseas stopped almost all use of mefloquine in malaria-prone areas in Africa and the Middle East. Army Col. Carol Labadie, the service's pharmacy program manager, commented on the long overdue change: "If that means changing from one drug to another because now this original drug has shown to be potentially harmful… it is in our interests to make that change."

As Croft wrote, it was not a case of inconvenient research being deliberately witheld. Rather, "the necessary pre-licensing research was simply never carried out."

Questions still remain about the use of mefloquine at Guantanamo as an "enhanced interrogation technique." **Last year, *Stars and Stripe*s ran an investigation of the matter and concluded: "Medical experts say the Defense Department policy of giving detainees large doses of mefloquine is poor medical practice at best and torture at worst."**

INTERVIEW WITH DR. REMINGTON NEVIN

——Is there any good science behind the notion that mefloquine might be addictive?

Dr. Remington Nevin: I am speaking to you in an individual capacity, and my opinions are my own and in no way reflect those of the U.S. Army or the Defense Department. There is no evidence that mefloquine is addictive per se, but the drug is well-known to produce vivid, technicolor dreams, and as a result it is frequently viewed as an incidental and convenient form of recreation among people, including Peace Corps volunteers and military service members, who find themselves already required to take the drug, and otherwise typically without access to alternative drugs of abuse, such as alcohol. The vivid "rock star" fantasies frequently reported are often perceived as consolation for the isolation and loneliness that typical accompany travel to remote areas where mefloquine is prescribed.

Ann Patchett, a prize-winning author, recently wrote a book called *State of Wonder* in which mefloquine features prominently, and her writing was likely based to a good degree on her and her acquaintances' experiences with the drug. Patchett herself actually refers to the drug's "recreational" properties and alludes in a recent interview to her having wanted to "take the drug out for a spin" (see http://thedianerehmshow.org/)

REHM: Did you take Lariam when you went to the Amazon?

PATCHETT: I did, I did. And actually, if I hadn't gone to the Amazon, I probably would've just taken it recreationally at home because I really wanted to take it out...

REHM: Experience it.

PATCHETT:...for a spin, right.

REHM: Yeah.

PATCHETT: And the side effects of Lariam listed on the package, psychotic dreams, terrible nightmares, paranoia, suicide is a possible side effect and I've known a lot of people who have had true psychosis on Lariam.

—Can you lay out what you know about mefloquine causing hallucinatory and dissociative effects in travelers who take it for malaria?

Dr. Nevin: [The symptoms] closely mimic those of a condition known as anti-NMDA receptor encephalitis, which an expert in the field, Dr. Dalmau, describes as including "anxiety, fear, bizarre or stereotypical behaviour, insomnia, and memory deficits". It is thought that rising levels of antibody to the NMDA receptor induces... widespread downstream dysregulation of limbic dopaminergic and noradrenergic tone, which ultimately are responsible for producing the syndrome's psychotic effects... This limbic dysregulation may also be similar to what is seen with the chemical NMDA receptor antagonists, including ketamine and phencyclidine, which share with mefloquine a particular propensity towards impulsivity and dissociation. For these reasons I conclude that mefloquine should be characterized as a dissociative hallucinogen.

—What is a dissociative hallucinogen?

Dr. Nevin: It is this property that also likely explains the drug's association with suicidality and acts of violence. Mefloquine is the only non-psychotropic drug listed among the top ten associated with acts of violence, and there is a growing literature linking it causally to suicide. It may be that the combination of mefloquine-induced amnesia, dissociation, and hallucinations (many with vivid religious or persecutory themes) creates a perfect storm that can trigger impulsive acts of violence. It is not uncommon for those recovering from (and surviving) mefloquine psychosis to report engaging in suicidal gestures that in retrospect were devoid of any fear of consequences.... Just within the past year, in a paper in the journal *Science*, Bissiere and colleagues demonstrated mefloquine interfering with context fear response in the hippocampus.

—*Could you expand on the notion of "vivid rock star fantasies" experienced by some users?*

Dr. Nevin: Extremely vivid dreams are among the most widely reported "adverse effect" of the drug. Users can frequently describe their dreams in great detail even well into the next day and, in some cases, the dreams seem to take on an almost lucid quality. Many experience gratifying and deeply pleasurable dreams that they almost don't wish to awaken from; conversely, for some others, the effect seems to be quite the opposite, with the reported nightmares being particularly haunting the next day.

—*You have referred to Lariam as a "zombie" drug. Could you expand on that?*

Dr. Nevin: If you must know, the reporter for *AP* caught me on Halloween, but I believe the term is quite apropos. The drug is the pharmaceutical equivalent of the living dead; it is somehow able to survive controversies that would have quickly killed other drugs. Interestingly, Lariam has been quietly delisted although generics remain widely available. To further stretch the metaphor, the drug is also decidedly neurotoxic and kills brain cells; one can say it "eats brains", and lastly, I would argue that a "zombie-like" state is not an unreasonable description of the most extreme adverse effects of the drug.

—I'm shocked to discover mefloquine on the list of top 10 drugs associated with acts of violence. Could you comment on a non-psychoactive drug making that list?

Dr. Nevin: It is quite shocking. Mefloquine isn't typically considered a psychotropic drug, but it probably should be recharacterized as a psychotropic medication with incidental anti-malarial properties. Of the drug contained in a 250mg tablet, only about 1-2mg, less than 1%, is ultimately found at the site of its intended anti-malarial activity, in the circulation. And although the neuropharmacokinetics are still somewhat unclear, arguably a far greater percentage of the drug is ultimately found in brain tissue than in the circulation. Incredibly, when the drug was undergoing FDA licensing, this brain penetration wasn't even well-characterized. Transcripts from the licensing meetings clearly show committee members skipping over this fact without much consideration. Certainly there seems to have been no requirement to submit the drug to neurotoxicity testing, despite many related quinoline compounds having demonstrated well-characterized, permanent neurotoxicity at least 40 years earlier.

—How common is the use of mefloquine in the U.S. as a whole?

Dr. Nevin: There has been a fairly rapid decline in the use of the drug, correlating with rising appreciation of mefloquine's dangers and awareness of contraindications to its safe use. Malarone is now the predominant anti-malarial prescribed within a large network of U.S. travel clinics. The U.S. military, which developed the drug just over 40 years ago, recently prohibited the use of mefloquine as first-line agent, and has dramatically curtailed its use after research revealed the drug had been widely prescribed to service members with mental health contraindications. Recently, the U.S. Centers for Disease Control further clarified guidance against routine use of mefloquine in service members, conceding that use of mefloquine may "confound the diagnosis and management of post-traumatic stress disorder and traumatic brain injury".

—What are the consequences of mixing Lariam with alcohol?

Dr. Nevin: There is fairly good evidence from case reports that alcohol may potentiate the deleterious effects of mefloquine, but the mechanism remains controversial. It had been suspected that alcohol simply exerted an inhibitory effect on mefloquine metabolism, but now… it seems likely that alcohol exerts a direct pharmacodynamic effect.

—Lariam is still sometimes prescribed for children traveling in malaria zones. Are there special dangers for kids?

Dr. Nevin: As the popularity of the drug is declining among adults, some experts with ties to industry have been peddling the drug for niche pediatric use, ostensibly because it is well tolerated. Unfortunately, such claims are based on studies which in many cases are deeply flawed and…. even verbally fluent but younger children may not have the experience or perspective to properly describe these symptoms. Apart from these considerations, I would argue that I don't think enough is understood about the neurophysiological effects of the drug to justify its use even in older children and adolescents. Mefloquine is a psychotropic drug. Given what we are learning of mefloquine's effects on the limbic system, even at relatively low doses, it seems at least plausible that the developing brain might in some way be adversely affected by the drug, particularly during long-term dosing.

—Why was the Army so slow to move on mefloquine?

Dr. Nevin: To put things in perspective, understand that mefloquine is the sole product of an aggressive 20-year, multi-million dollar effort by the U.S. Army. Mefloquine was identified only in the early 1970s after tens of thousands of other quinoline compounds had failed toxicity and efficacy tests. By the time of mefloquine's U.S. licensure in 1989, it was essentially DoD's last and only hope. So, if I could rephrase your question, if mefloquine is as safe as the Army once claimed, then why is it no longer the drug of choice? If we assume that this quiet policy change was made in tacit acknowledge of safety concerns, then the question is, precisely what new information has informed this decision, why has this change taken so long to occur, and most importantly, what harm might this policy change now be seeking to avoid, which may already have accrued among those in whom the drug had been previously used?

The reasons for the Army's silence on these questions are likely quite banal. Admitting mefloquine is a dangerous drug would be a bitter pill for any Army medical leader to swallow. Many of today's senior medical leaders were intimately involved in the studies that saw the drug rise to prominence, and many are on record over the previous decades publicly defending the drug against the increasingly validated claims of its earlier critics. Absent external pressure to do so, it is likely of little benefit for these senior medical leaders to suffer the humiliation that would come from admitting what they might now otherwise privately concede. Saying nothing is the path of least resistance on their journey to a comfortable retirement.

—*Could you comment on allegations of Lariam use as an interrogation drug at Guantanamo?*

Dr. Nevin: The use of mefloquine at Guantanamo represents either medical malpractice with culpability at some of the highest levels of military medical leadership, or it suggests something far more intentional and sinister. I typically believe that one should never ascribe to malice what can be attributed to simple incompetence, but in this case, I am not so certain. There are too many inconsistencies and unanswered questions. The issue will ultimately require the release of medical records, open hearings, and testimony to resolve. I am confident this will happen.

Monday, February 6, 2012

http://addiction-dirkh.blogspot.com/2012/02/
army-doctor-sees-victory-and-dangerous.html

Moderate Drinking:
The Debate Continues

New study says it's the lifestyle, not the alcohol.

Ever since the first studies showed modest statistical health benefits for people who drank a light to moderate amount of alcohol, the debate has bounced back and forth among researchers. Now an Italian study of more than 3,000 older adults, published in the *Journal of the American Geriatrics Society*, claims that it is the moderate lifestyle of drinkers, and not the alcohol itself, which helps prevent functional decline as we age.

After controlling for body weight, level of physical activity, education, and income, Cinzia Maraldi and coworkers in the Department of Clinical and Experimental Internal Medicine at the University of Ferrara pointed the finger at lifestyle characteristics—primarily weight control and exercise.

The researchers did not dispute the finding that moderate levels of alcohol intake can lower the risk of cardiovascular diseas— but lead author Maraldi said in a press release that "the benefit of alcohol intake on other health-related outcomes is less convincing."

Maraldi said the positive effects of moderate alcohol on physical aging and cognitive impairment in the elderly may be only apparent, "because life-style related characteristics seem to be the real determinant of the reported association."

The research follows earlier U.S. studies suggesting much the same thing. A finding that had become common folk wisdom—with perhaps a little nudge from the alcoholic beverage industry—is now openly disputed by scientists.

"The moderate drinkers tend to do everything right," said sociologist Kaye Middleton Fillmore, in a *New York Times* article by Roni Caryn Rabin. "They exercise, they don't smoke, they eat right and they drink moderately." In the same article, an Oakland cardiologist said: "It's very difficult to form a single-bullet message because one size doesn't fit all here, and the public health message has to be very conservative."

In the *New York Times* article, Dr. Tim Naimi of the Centers for Disease Control and Prevention said: **"The bottom line is there has not been a single study done on moderate alcohol consumption and mortality outcomes that is a 'gold standard' kind of study**—the kind of randomized controlled clinical trial that we would be required to have in order to approve a new pharmaceutical agent in this country."

Sunday, October 18, 2009

http://addiction-dirkh.blogspot.com/2009/10/moderate-drinking-debate-continues.html

Personalizing Addiction Medicine

Gene variants make anti-craving drugs a hit-or-miss affair.

Rather than taking on another broad hunt for the genes controlling the expression of alcoholism, noted addiction researcher Dr. Bankole Johnson and co-workers at the Department of Psychiatry and Neurobehavioral Sciences at the University of Virginia took a different tack. **The researchers focused, instead, on investigating whether genetic variations among alcoholics might affect their responses to a specific anti-craving medication.**

The result, according to Kenneth Warren, acting director of the National Institute on Alcohol Abuse and Alcoholism (NIAAA), is a study that represents "an important milestone in the search for personalized treatments for alcohol dependence."

For any addiction, once it has been active for a sustained period, the first-line treatment of the future is likely to be biological. New addiction treatments will come—and in many cases already do come—in the form of drugs to treat drug addiction. **Every day, addicts are quitting drugs and alcohol by availing themselves of drug treatments that did not exist fifteen years ago.** As more of the biological substrate is teased out, the search for effective approaches narrows along avenues that are more fruitful. This is the most promising, and, without doubt, the most controversial development in the history of addiction treatment.

The researchers were interested in variations in the gene controlling the expression of a serotonin transporter protein. Dr. Johnson's earlier work had centered on teasing out the influence the serotonin 5-HTT transporter exerts on the development of alcoholism. Previous research had focused attention on the so-called LL and TT variants of this transporter gene. After performing genetic analyses to determine which test subjects were carrying which versions of the gene in question, Dr. Johnson and his colleagues conducted a controlled trial of ondansetron on a randomized group of 283 alcoholics.

The findings were published in the *American Journal of Psychiatry*.

Ondansetron is an anti-emetic medication that has shown promise in treating addictions, particularly alcoholism. Ondansetron (trade name Zofran), helps block the nausea of chemotherapy by altering serotonin activity in the GI tract. (Vomiting is a serotonin-mediated reflex.) **The scientists found that "individuals with the LL geno-type who received ondansetron had a lower mean number of drinks per day (-1.62) and a higher percentage of days abstinent (11.27%) than those who received placebo."** This put the ondansetron drinkers under five drinks a day. All of the placebo drinkers continued to exceed the five drinks per day mark.

But the strongest difference was found in the group of alcoholics who possessed both the LL and TT genetic variants. **The LL/TT alcoholics taking ondansetron "had a lower number of drinks per drinking day (-2.63) and a higher percentage of days abstinent (16.99%) than all other geno-type and treatment groups combined."**

The goal here is straightforward. In an email exchange, Dr. Johnson told me: "I agree that it would be great if we could use a pharmacogenetic approach to study other anti-craving drugs. The idea of providing the right drug to the right person is definitely important for optimizing therapeutic effects and minimizing side-effects."

It won't be easy. Such genetic testing is still in its infancy, and complications abound. For example, in an earlier study in the *Journal of the American Medical Association*, Dr. Johnson found that diagnosed patients who received ondansetron over an 11-week period increased their days of abstinence compared to alcoholics on placebo. However, in that study, **"The researchers found no differences between ondansetron patients with late-onset alcoholism and those who received placebo."** This suggests that, along with genetic variations, ondansetron's effectiveness with alcoholics may also depend on the type of alcoholism under consideration: early onset or late onset.

We have a long way to go, but individualized pharmaceutical assistance in the early stages of addiction recovery remains the Holy Grail for many addiction researchers. And hopes are running high.

Friday, January 21, 2011

http://addiction-dirkh.blogspot.com/2011/01/
personalizing-addiction-medicine.html

Johnson, B., Ait-Daoud, N., Seneviratne, C., Roache, J., Javors, M., Wang, X., Liu, L., Penberthy, J., DiClemente, C., & Li, M. Pharmacogenetic Approach at the Serotonin Transporter Gene as a Method of Reducing the Severity of Alcohol Drinking *American Journal of Psychiatry* 2011. DOI: 10.1176/appi.ajp.2010.10050755

What is Methadone?

How agonists ease agony for heroin addicts.

It isn't the best, the worst, or the only treatment for heroin addiction. But for many heroin addicts, it has been a way out of the circle of euphoria and dispair.

In contrast to antagonist drugs, the agonist theory is based on drugs that bind to specific sites and which mimic some of the addictive drug's typical range of effects. For obvious reasons, this greatly reduces craving. But is it simply a replay of the historical tactic of substituting one addictive drug for another?

The most successful use of the agonist theory remains heroin's most controversial and stigmatized treatment—methadone therapy. Back in the 1960s, researchers at Rockefeller Hospital and The Rockefeller Institute, led by Professor Vincent Dole of Rockefeller University, began a series of studies that led to the development of methadone treatment. They did it on the strength of their belief in the unfolding biological model. "Heroin addiction is a disease of the brain, with diverse physical and behavioral ramifications, and not simply due to criminal behavior, a personality disorder, or 'weak will,'" wrote Dr. Kreek, one of the principle methadone researchers at Rockefeller.

Methadone was approved by the FDA in 1973 for medical use against heroin addiction. It is a slow-acting opiate receptor agonist, meaning that it has some of the properties of heroin and morphine. However, the buzz it provides is no real substitute for heroin or morphine, from an addict's point of view. It was nobody's idea of a sweet drug holiday. But why give agonist drugs to addicts at all? Isn't that just like giving them watered-down heroin? Writing in the September 2002 issue of *Nature Reviews Drug Discovery*, Dr. Kreek summed up what doctors face when dealing with long-term addiction:

"Repeated 'on-off' exposure to a drug of abuse progressively leads to stable molecular and cellular changes in neurons, which alter the activity of neural networks that contain these neurons. This eventually results in complex physiological changes and related behaviors that characterize addiction, such as tolerance, sensitization, dependence, withdrawal, craving and stress-induced relapse. These drug-induced changes are, in part, counter-adaptive, and they contribute to dysphoria and dysfunction, which promotes continued drug use through negative-reinforcement mechanisms."

Daily methadone doses of 80mg or more exert a definite blocking effect on heroin craving. And patients who use it do not suffer the same lassitude and intensity of cognitive distortions as the heroin addict. **Methadone's other strength is that it doesn't mix well with heroin or alcohol.**

More recently, Kreek and her colleagues, in collaboration with the NIH, used PET scans to watch opioid-receptor binding occur in the living brains of methadone-maintained patients. The brain scans confirmed that methadone leaves a significant number of opioid receptors unoccupied, allowing those regions of the brain to carry out normal physiological roles.

"In methadone-maintained patients there is modest occupancy of the receptors but still a lot of available receptors for normal cognition, normal reproductive function and normal stress responsivity," Kreek reported.

Another underreported advantage of methadone is its oral administration, thus eliminating the need for hypodermics and reducing the risk of AIDS and hepatitis

from contaminated needles. Provided the dosage is right, patients can be maintained for years on methadone. One reason methadone therapy fails, say researchers, is because of inadequate dosages—but higher dosages are much harder to withdraw from.

Thursday, August 12, 2010

http://addiction-dirkh.blogspot.com/2010/08/what-is-methadone.html

The Future of Addiction Treatment

Is there some way out of here?

Addictions are chronic diseases. They may require a lifetime of treatment. After a number of severe episodes of alcohol or drug abuse, the brain may be organically primed for more of the same. Long-term treatment is sometimes, if not always, the most effective way out of this dilemma. (The same is true of unipolar depression.)

We will need to learn a lot more about chemicals—the ones we ingest, and the ones that are produced and stored naturally in our bodies—if we plan to make any serious moves toward more effective treatment. What we have learned about the nature of pleasure and reward is a strong start. **The guiding insight behind most of the work is that addiction to different drugs involves reward and pleasure mechanisms common to them all. The effects of the drug—whether it makes you sleepy, stimulated, happy, talkative, or delusional—constitute a secondary phenomenon.** A good deal of earlier research was directed at teasing out the customized peculiarities of one drug of abuse compared to another. Now most addiction scientists agree that receptor alterations in response to the artificial stimulation produced by the drugs are the biochemical key, and that recovery occurs when the brain's remarkable "plastic" abilities go to work at the molecular level, re-regulating and adjusting to the new, drug-free or drug-reduced status quo. An addict beats addiction by ceasing the constant and artificial

205

manipulation of neuronal receptors, to be entirely unromantic for a moment about the nature of recovery.

But in order for that to happen most effectively, you have to stop taking the drugs.

Comparing our reservoir of pleasure chemicals to money in the bank, Dr. George Koob, Chairman of the Committee On The Neurobiology Of Addictive Disorders at the Scripps Institute in La Jolla, California, draws the following analogy:

We can expend that money over the course of a single weekend's binge on cocaine or we can expend it over a two-week period in the normal pleasures of everyday life. If you spend these pleasure neurochemicals in one lump sum such as a crack binge, you use up your supply of pleasure for a certain period, and so you pay for it later.

Addicts vividly demonstrate a compulsive need to use alcohol and other drugs despite the worst kinds of consequences—arrest, illness, injury, overdose. What kind of euphoria could be worth such psychic pain? Even stranger, why continue when the drug no longers works as well as it once did due to tolerance? **What makes these people eat their words, shred their best intentions, break their promises, and starting using or drinking again and again?**

There really is no cheating in this game. The system has to self-regulate. Craving and drug-seeking behavior, once set in motion, disrupt an individual's normal "motivational hierarchy." How does this motivational express train come about? It happens at the point where casual experimentation is replaced by the pharmacological dictates of active addiction. It happens when the impulse to try it with your friends transforms itself into the drug-hungry monkey on your back.

Formal medical treatment and intervention *can* work, but the results are inconsistent and often little better than no formal treatment at all. **Most alcoholics and smokers and other drug addicts, it is frequently asserted, become abstinent on their own, going through detoxification, withdrawal,**

and subsequent cravings without benefit of any formal programs. Our health policy should not only encourage addicts to heal themselves, but must also help equip them with the medical tools they need in treatment. After all, behavioral habits as relatively harmless as nail biting can be all but impossible to break.

As detailed by Dr. Mary Jeanne Kreek, a professor and senior attending physician at the Laboratory of the Biology of Addictive Diseases at Rockefeller University:

Toxicity, destruction of previously formed synapses, formation of new synapses, enhancement or reduction of cognition and the development of specific memories of the drug of abuse, which are coupled with the conditioned cues for enhancing relapse to drug use, all have a role in addiction. And each of these provides numerous potential targets for pharmacotherapies for the future.

In other words, when an addiction has been active for a sustained period, the first-line treatment of the future is likely to come in the form of a pill. New addiction treatments will come—and in many cases already do come—in the form of drugs to treat drug addiction. **Every day, addicts are quitting drugs and alcohol by availing themselves of pharmaceutical treatments that did not exist twenty years ago. Sometimes medications work, and we all need to reacquaint ourselves with that notion.** As more of the biological substrate is teased out, the search for effective medications narrows along more fruitful avenues.

Fighting fire with fire is not without risk, of course. None of this is meant to deny the usefulness of talk therapy as an adjunct to treatment. However, consider the risks involved in *not* finding more effective medical treatments. Better addiction treatment is, by almost any measure, a cost-effective proposition.

Sunday, February 12, 2012

http://addiction-dirkh.blogspot.com/2012/02/future-of-addiction-treatment.html

Why Drug Stigma Still Matters

More sinned against than sinning?

"Psychological theories of illness are a powerful means of placing the blame on the ill. Patients who are instructed that they have, unwittingly, caused their disease are also being made to feel that they have deserved it."

—Susan Sontag, *Illness as Metaphor*

Addiction is always a hot topic, in its way, if only because of an endless supply of fallible starlets. More seriously, valuable research is taking place in myriad directions—the psychology of addiction, the disease of addiction, the neurobiology of addiction, the neuropsychopharmacology of addiction, etc. What sometimes goes missing is any serious analysis of the stigmatization of drug addiction.

The UK Drug Policy Commission (UKDPC) is an independent research group comprised of 12 "expert commissioners" charged with providing objective analysis on drug policy matters. The group issued a paper authored by Charlie Lloyd of the University of York. In "Sinning and Sinned Against: The Stigmatisation of Problem Drug Users," Lloyd set out to pull together the evidence-based research on the effects of stigmatizing "problem drug users." The European Monitoring Centre for Drugs and Drug Addiction (EMCDDA) defines problem drug use as "injecting drug use or long-duration/ regular use of opioids, cocaine and/or amphetamines."

According to Lloyd's analysis of the research literature, the groups most frequently referred to as stigmatized are the disabled, the mentally ill, minority ethnic groups—and drug addicts. To make matters worse, multiple problems often attach to addicts:

"Problem drug users frequently report suffering from other stigmas: being black, female, Hepatitis C or HIV positive, disabled, or suffering from a mental disorder. However, research shows that problem drug user status is the most stigmatising." The stigma is continuously cemented in place by rhetoric about the "war on drugs." There is no comparable public war on disability, or mental illness, or ethnicity—at least not overtly.

I cannot vouch for Lloyd's analysis, but a good deal of it smacks of common sense at the street level. Others have suggested it is logical to assume that the stigma attached to hard drug addiction serves, by example, to deter others. "However," Lloyd writes, "attempts to scare young people away from drug use have not proved effective. The evidence reviewed here suggests that stigma keeps users away from treatment."

So this is not a theoretical concern. Stigmatization "may be a major stumbling block to successful rehabilitation." Health professionals and hospital staff "can be distrustful and judgmental in dealing with problem drug users but drug users can themselves be aggressive and manipulative. In the United States staff who choose to work in hospitals serving the most deprived, inner-city populations appear to be more compassionate and patient."

The prevailing public view, Lloyd writes, is that problem drug users tend to be "dangerous, deceitful, unreliable, unpredictable, hard to talk with and to blame for their predicament. Young people may have more negative views in this respect than adults."

Of course, drug addicts can be all those things at one time or another. Drug abusers often stigmatize themselves. For the user, these conflicted feelings lead some of them to feel that "the very act of seeking treatment serves to cement an 'addict' or 'junkie' identity, which can lead to further rejection from family and friends."

This is most commonly experienced by users on methadone maintenance treatment, "who feel particularly stigmatised, in comparison to other treatment types." Lloyd notes that a lifetime stigma sometimes attaches to heroin and cocaine addiction, continuing "to haunt such ex-users, preventing access to good housing and employment." As he trenchantly observes, there is plenty of room "to stigmatise users less, without rendering heroin or crack-cocaine significantly more attractive."

Lloyd concludes that the primary culprit, the complicating factor, is "blame." Compared to "blameless groups" such as the disabled and the mentally ill, problem drug users, he writes, "are blamed for taking drugs in the first place and are also perceived to have a choice whether or not to take drugs in the future."

If public and professional stigma has the power to prevent addicts from entering treatment (as it formerly held a similar power over the mentally ill, and before that, the disabled), what can be done about it? Lloyd makes several concrete suggestions, most of which center, predictably, on education:

Drug education in schools should focus on the causes and the consequences of active addiction, rather than relying on scare stories.

—It's time to teach health care and pharmacy staff about the medical, social, and psychological aspects of drug addiction.

—Treatment agencies need to focus on the whole person, "and not see problem drug users as solely problem drug users. Some drug addicts are also bird-watchers."

—Users themselves, as well as their families, often benefit from a greater understanding of the mechanisms of addiction. This can have the effect of reducing "the self-blame felt by many drug user's parents."

—Finally, "police need to reflect on their practice in policing problem drug users at street level." 'Nuff said on that.

DrugScope, a leading U.K. charity with a membership drawn in part from the ranks of drug treatment and education workers, praised the report as "timely and insightful." Martin Barnes, chief executive of DrugScope, said that the report effectively "evidences stigma as a barrier to recovery and reintegration."

Saturday, September 4, 2010

http://addiction-dirkh.blogspot.com/2010/09/why-drug-stigma-still-matters.htm

The "Broken Bone" Model of Addiction Treatment

A word about chronic illnesses.

It's not always easy to conceive of addiction as a complex disease—but it's getting easier. There are certain similarities among chronic diseases. As with diabetes, asthma, and high blood pressure, drug addiction often requires protracted and multi-faceted treatments—treatments that typically do not produce the kinds of dramatic cures and breakthroughs that are associated with recovery from other kinds of medical conditions.

As we become increasingly comfortable with the concept of addictive disease, we risk losing sight of a crucial distinction between *acute* medical disorders, like infections and broken bones; and *chronic* disorders with multiple biological, psychological, and social components, like diabetes and addiction.

William L. White of Chestnut Health Systems, and Thomas McClellan, Executive Director of the Treatment Research Institute and former deputy director of the Office of National Drug Control Policy (ONDCP) in the White House, co-authored a paper for *Counselor Magazine* that seeks to make the distinction clear. In "Addiction as a Chronic Disorder," the two seasoned treatment professionals point out that "chronic care has to be quite different from acute care," and that all treatments for chronic diseases like diabetes and addiction have three things in common:

1) They reduce symptoms but cannot affect root causes. Such treatments "do not return the affected individual to normal."

2) They require major changes in lifestyle and behavior for maximum effectiveness. **For example, "even if individuals with diabetes regularly take their insulin as prescribed, this will not stop disease progression if they do not also reduce sugar and starch intake, increase exercise and reduce stress levels."**

3) Due to their complex nature, "relapses are likely to occur in all chronic illnesses. Increasingly, family members are being trained to also provide continued monitoring, " the authors point out.

So far, so good. But chronic care treatment is not what addiction treatment in America is really about. **Addiction treatment in both medical and private settings is frequently governed by acute care thinking—the "broken bone" model of treatment.** For example:

—"Services are delivered 'programmatically' in a uniform series of encapsulated activities (screen admission, a single point-in-time assessment, treatment procedures, discharge, brief 'aftercare' followed by termination of the service relationship)."

—"Services transpire over a short (and historically ever-shorter) period of time, usually as a function of pre-arranged, time-limited insurance payments."

—"The individual/family/community is given the impression at discharge ('graduation') that 'cure has occurred.'"

—"Post-treatment relapse and re-admissions are viewed as the failure (non-compliance) of the individual rather than potential flaws in the design or execution of the treatment protocol."

Some fifteen years ago, the acute care model began to fall under increasing scrutiny as the neurosciences took wing and insights related to chronic diseases of the body and brain began to accumulate. **As White and McClellan are at pains to point out,**

heavy drinking and other forms of drug abuse do not inexorably become chronic disorders. "Many substance use problems are developmental and as such are often outgrown in the successful transition from adolescence into adulthood. Others occur in tandem with major life transitions (e.g., death of a loved one, divorce, job loss) and are resolved by time, natural support, brief professional intervention or peer-based intervention by others in recovery."

It's the same with high blood pressure: A period of hypertension may or may not lead to a chronic condition, and at present it's difficult to predict whose high blood pressure is likely to prove resistant to changes in diet, exercise, and weight.

Beyond the matter of treatment, what do chronic diseases like asthma, diabetes, and addiction really have in common?

—They are influenced by both genetic and environmental risk factors.

—They have "a prolonged course that varies from person to person in intensity and pattern."

—They are accompanied by "risks of profound pathophysiology, disability and premature death."

—They have effective treatments, and "similar remission rates, but no known cures."

If substance dependence is like other chronic illnesses, then two important insights follow: 1) "Acute care models of intervention for severe substance dependence may reduce substance use temporarily but those reductions are not likely to sustain once care stops," and 2) "methods used in the treatment of other chronic illnesses might be effectively adapted to enhance long-term recovery from substance dependence."

In the end, the authors argue that acute forms of treatment applied to a chronic disorder "offer an explanation of the generally high and rapid rates of relapse following cessation of most available addiction treatments: there is simply no quick fix for the most severe forms of this disorder."

Sunday, March 13, 2011

http://addiction-dirkh.blogspot.com/2011/03/broken-bone-model-of-addiction.html

Rethinking the Patch

Quitters do better on 6-month regimen.

It may sound like dream propaganda for the makers of nicotine patches. And it is. Moreover, at least one of the study authors has worked in the past as a consultant for GlaxoSmithKline, maker of Nicoderm CQ, one of the best-selling brands of transdermal nicotine patches.

So there is every reason to dismiss a 2010 study by researchers at the University of Pennsylvania School of Medicine, published in the *Annals of Internal Medicine*, which strongly suggests that the currently recommended regimen of two months isn't long enough. It should be tripled. Which would also triple sales.

There's only one catch: There is reason to believe that the results are legitimate, and that smokers who are trying to quit would be more successful if they stuck with the patch for longer periods than currently recommended on the manufacturer's box. **For some time now, tobacco addiction researchers, and centers such as Mayo Clinic's Stop Smoking facilities, have recognized the need for extending the manufacturer's suggested period of use.**

Referring to the patch on its Stop Smoking web site, Mayo Clinic says: "You typically use the nicotine patch for eight to 12 weeks. You may need to use it longer if cravings or withdrawal symptoms continue."

And from the field come reports of abstaining smokers independently choosing to use the patch

longer, often by cutting the patches into eighths or sixteenths in order to accomplish a long, slow taper at the end of the process. By following this route, a nicotine addict need not be aware of the precise day or moment when his nicotine fix from the patch has dropped to placebo levels—further evidence that nicotine addiction is a chronic condition that may not respond to treatments of only two to three months in duration.

One early development during the marketing of the patch that helped set the short-term use pattern were reports in the 1990s of heart attacks by patch users. **Subsequent research showed that rare cardiac problems had arisen in patients who had continued heavy smoking while on the patch, and that there was little evidence of a direct link between nicotine patches and heart attacks.** (Recent heart attack victims are advised to wait six weeks and use patches with caution.)

The study concludes: "Transdermal nicotine for 24 weeks increased biochemically confirmed point-prevalence abstinence and continuous abstinence at week 24, reduced the risk for smoking lapses, and increased the likelihood of recovery to abstinence after a lapse compared with 8 weeks of transdermal nicotine therapy."

One limitation of this particular study, acknowledged as such by the authors, is that "participants were smokers without medical comorbid conditions who were seeking treatment." In other words, the study cohort consisted of highly motivated smokers.

And another problem is cost: Few health insurance companies cover the full cost of patches, including Medicaid. **The additional cost per quitter, the study found, was about $2,400 for the extended regimen.**

Nonetheless, any uptick in success rates for smoking cessation programs should be noted and taken under consideration.

Sunday, February 7, 2010

http://addiction-dirkh.blogspot.com/2010/02/rethinking-patch.html

Robert A. Schnoll, PhD; Freda Patterson, PhD; E. Paul Wileyto, PhD; Daniel F. Heitjan, PhD; Alexandra E. Shields, PhD; David A. Asch, MD; and Caryn Lerman, PhD. Effectiveness of Extended-Duration Transdermal Nicotine Therapy: A Randomized Trial *Annals of Internal Medicine*. 152(3):144-151. 2010.

Marijuana Withdrawal

For Some Users, Cannabis Can Be Fiercely Addictive.

For a minority of marijuana users, commonly estimated at 10 per cent, the use of pot can become uncontrollable, as with any other addictive drug. Addiction to marijuana is frequently submerged in the welter of polyaddictions common to active addicts. The withdrawal rigors of, say, alcohol or heroin tend to drown out the subtler, more psychological manifestations of cannabis withdrawal.

What has emerged in the past ten years is a profile of marijuana withdrawal, where none existed before. The syndrome is marked by irritability, restlessness, generalized anxiety, hostility, depression, difficulty sleeping, excessive sweating, loose stools, loss of appetite, and a general "blah" feeling. **Many patients complain of feeling like they have a low-grade flu, and they describe a psychological state of existential uncertainty—"inner unrest," as one researcher calls it.**

The most common marijuana withdrawal symptom is low-grade anxiety. Anxiety of this sort has a firm biochemical substrate, produced by withdrawal, craving, and detoxification from almost all drugs of abuse. It is not the kind of anxiety that can be deflected by forcibly thinking "happy thoughts," or staying busy all the time.

A peptide known as corticotrophin-releasing factor (CRF) is linked to this kind of anxiety. Neurologists at the Scripps Research Institute in La Jolla, California, noting that anxiety is the universal keynote symptom of drug and alcohol withdrawal, started looking at the release of CRF in the amygdala. After documenting elevated CRF levels in rat brains during alcohol, heroin, and cocaine withdrawal, the researchers injected synthetic THC into 50 rats once a day for two weeks. (For better or worse, this is how many of the animal models simulate heavy, long-term pot use in humans). Then they gave the rats a THC agonist that bound to the THC receptors without activating them. The result: The rats exhibited withdrawal symptoms such as compulsive grooming and teeth chattering—the kinds of stress behaviors rats engage in when they are kicking the habit. In the end, when the scientists measured CRF levels in the amygdalas of the animals, they found three times as much CRF, compared to animal control groups.

While subtler and more drawn out, the process of kicking marijuana can now be demonstrated as a neurochemical fact. **It appears that marijuana increases dopamine and serotonin levels through the intermediary activation of opiate and GABA receptors.** Drugs like naloxone, which block heroin, might have a role to play in marijuana detoxification.

As Dr. DeChiara of the Italian research team suggested in *Science*, "this overlap in the effects of THC and opiates on the reward pathway may provide a biological basis for the controversial 'gateway hypothesis,' in which smoking marijuana is thought to cause some people to abuse harder drugs." America's second favorite drug, De Chiara suggests, may prime the brain to seek substances like heroin. In rebuttal, marijuana experts Lester Grinspoon and James Bakalar of Harvard Medical school have protested this resumed interest in the gateway theory, pointing out that if substances that boost dopamine in the reward pathways are gateways to heroin use, than we had better add chocolate, sex, and alcohol to the list.

In the end, what surprised many observers was simply that the idea of treatment for marijuana dependence seemed to appeal to such a large number of people. The Addiction Research Foundation in Toronto has reported that even brief interventions, in the form of support group sessions, can be useful for addicted pot smokers.

In 2005, an article in the *American Journal of Psychiatry* concluded that, for patients recently out of rehab, "**Postdischarge cannabis use substantially and significantly increased the hazard of first use of any substance** and strongly reduced the likelihood of stable remission from use of any substance."

Wednesday, October 17, 2007

http://addiction-dirkh.blogspot.com/2007/10/marijuana-withdrawal.html

Acupuncture for Addiction: It Doesn't Look Good

Needles fail in latest study of opiate detox.

Acupuncture as a treatment for drug addiction took another punch recently in a study published in the *Journal of Substance Abuse Treatment*. In "Auricular acupuncture as an adjunct to opiate detoxification treatment," the study authors investigated whether acupuncture would "add value" to a standard methadone-based detoxification process. For the two-week study, 82 opiate-addicted patients were randomly assigned to either ear acupuncture by qualified acupuncturists, or the attachment of ear clips by non-professionals. Each day, the study participants were tested for withdrawal severity and craving.

"On none of the 14 days," the authors report, "were there statistically significant differences between patients allocated to 'real' acupuncture and the 'sham' treatment. Such statistically insignificant difference as there were favored the 'sham' treatment...."

The results, say the authors, "are consistent with the findings of other studies which failed to find any effect of acupuncture in the treatment of drug dependence." Moreover, the authors conclude, this finding is "particularly disappointing as if anything the circumstances favored the acupuncture option," since in contrast "the alternative may not have been seen as a convincing therapy."

Nevertheless, **"like the featured study, previous studies of acupuncture in the treatment of opiate addiction have been unconvincing....** The 'ineffective' verdict on acupuncture extends to the treatment of cocaine dependence," the authors maintain, while an attempt to replicate earlier positive findings on acupuncture for alcohol dependence found no benefits, either.

The authors also reflect on whether such offerings, though of dubious value, attract addicts to treatment centers. "The possibility remains that offering something concrete like acupuncture helps attract people to services, and that doing something both clients and staff believe is worthwhile (even if it is a 'sham' procedure) helps retain patients in treatment, and in doing so improves outcomes."

Of course, this is only one study out of many, and acupuncture enthusiasts remain as optimistic as ever. Proponents of acupuncture treatment **continue to petition the National Institute on Drug Abuse (NIDA) for endorsement.** Most reports of success remain anecdotal. Nonetheless, the National Acupuncture Detoxification Association estimates that there are 200 acupuncture detoxification programs operating in the United States and Europe.

Tuesday, May 5, 2009

http://addiction-dirkh.blogspot.com/2009/05/acupuncture-for-addiction-it-doesnt.html

Auricular acupuncture as an adjunct to opiate detoxification treatment: effects on withdrawal symptoms. Bearn J., Swami A., Stewart D. et al. *Journal of Substance Abuse Treatment.* 36, 345–349. 2009.

Heroin for Heroin Addiction

Getting your fix at the doctor's office.

A group of Canadian researchers has demonstrated the truth of a practice commonly used in European countries like The Netherlands and Switzerland: Heroin can be an effective treatment for chronic, relapsing heroin addicts. Published in the *New England Journal of Medicine*, the study is "the first rigorous test of the approach performed in North America," according to a *New York Times* article by Benedict Carey.

In the study, 226 patients were randomly assigned to oral methadone therapy or injectable diacetylmorphine, the primary active ingredient in heroin, over a 12-month period. **The "rate of retention in addiction treatment" was 88 percent for the diacetylmorphine group, compared to 54 percent for the methadone group**. The "reduction in rates of illicit-drug use" was 67 percent for the heroin group and 48 percent for the methadone group.

Using doctor-prescribed heroin has two advantages, some researchers believe. It gets around the problem of addicts who don't like the effect of methadone and therefore don't take it as prescribed. Moreover, as European countries have demonstrated, it brings treatment-resistant opiate addicts into regular contact with physicians and medical treatment professionals, thereby keeping them away from drug dealers and out of jail.

The downside is equally obvious. It keeps addicts hooked on heroin, and may even exacerbate their addiction by providing a higher quality drug. Furthermore, it runs against the prevailing North American notion that heroin should be illegal, period. Certainly, doctors have no business prescribing it to active addicts, critics argue. Furthermore, the risk of overdose or seizure is always present.

According to senior author Martin Schechter of the University of British Columbia's School of Population and Public Health, as quoted in the *New York Times*: **"The main finding is that for this group that is generally written off, both methadone and prescription heroin can provide real benefits."**

In an editorial accompanying the journal article, Virginia Berridge of the London School of Hygiene and Tropical Medicine cautioned that "the rise and fall of methods of treatment in this controversial area owe their rationale to evidence, but they also often owe more to the politics of the situation."

At the end of the 19th Century in America, opium was widely prescribed as a cure for alcoholism. For opium addiction, the treatment was often alcohol.

Tuesday, August 25, 2009

http://addiction-dirkh.blogspot.com/2009/08/heroin-f
or-heroin-addiction.html

Treadmill Rehab

The curious connection between exercise and getting high.

A Vanderbilt study published in the journal *PLoS ONE* has confirmed what readers of Addiction Inbox have known for some time: Exercise often helps to curb cravings for addictive drugs. The Vanderbilt paper is noteworthy for focusing on heavy marijuana smokers (6 joints per day) who had not expressed any interest in quitting. Yet, at the end of a modest two-week exercise regimen, the participants reported less cannabis use.

Last August, I wrote about a growing body of research suggesting that the runner's high and the cannabis high were more similar than previously imagined. Investigators wired up college students, put them to work in a gym, and found that "exercise of moderate intensity dramatically increased concentrations of anandamide in blood plasma."

The *British Journal of Sports Medicine* ran a research review, "Endocannabinoids and exercise," which seriously disputed the "endorphin hypothesis" assumed to be behind the runner's high. The primary problem is that the opioid system is responsible for respiratory depression, pinpoint pupils, and other effects distinctly unhelpful to runners and other strenuous exercisers.

Compared to endorphins, the analgesia produced by the endocannabinoid system is much more consistent with the demands of exercise. Very high doses of marijuana tend to have a sedating effect, but low doses tend to induce activity or hyperactivity. There are cannabinoid receptors in muscles, skin, and the lungs. Moreover, "cannabinoids produce neither the respiratory depression, meiosis, or strong inhibition of gastrointestinal motility associated with opiates and opioids," according to the research review. "This is because there are few CB1 receptors in the brainstem and, apparently, the large intestine."

In addition, in my 2008 post entitled "Battling Addiction with Exercise," I highlighted director Nora Volkow's remarks at a NIDA-sponsored conference on addiction treatment and research: **"Exercise has been shown to be beneficial in so many areas of physical and mental health," Volkow said.** "This cross-disciplinary meeting is designed to get scientists thinking creatively about its potential role in substance abuse prevention."

At the same conference, Dr. Bess Marcus of Brown University, working on a NIDA-funded study of exercise for smoking cessation, presented the scientific evidence for the addiction/exercise connection. Similarities in the effects on the reward pathways of the brain's limbic system—dopamine activity in particular—may tie the two behaviors together more directly than previously thought. Among the findings:

—Rats in cages with running wheels show less interest in amphetamine infusions than rats without exercise options.

—Baby monkeys who don't roughhouse with their peers have higher levels of impulse control problems and alcohol use when they get older.

—In humans, exercise is known to reduce stress and tension—and anxiety is a well-known side effect of withdrawal, from alcohol and cigarettes to heroin and speed.

—Physical activity may enhance cellular growth in key areas of the brain involved in addiction, thereby aiding the neural changes that take place during detoxification and withdrawal from addictive drugs.

Tuesday, March 8, 2011

http://addiction-dirkh.blogspot.com/2011/03/treadmill-rehab.html

Buchowski MS, Meade NN, Charboneau E, Park S, Dietrich MS, et al. Aerobic Exercise Training Reduces Cannabis Craving and Use in Non-Treatment Seeking Cannabis-Dependent Adults. PLoS ONE 6(3): e17465. 2011. doi:10.1371/journal.pone.0017465

The Patch and How to Use It

Take the Fagerstrom test.

In 2009, the *U.K. Guardian*, in partnership with the *British Medical Journal*, offered its readers a short version of the Fagerstrom test, a questionnaire used for assessing the intensity of physical addiction to nicotine. The *Guardian* article then made recommendations about which patch strength smokers should be using, based on their scores.

Here is a longer version of the Fagerstrom test, with scoring assessment, followed by the Guardian's recommendations about patches:

Fagerstrom Test for Nicotine Dependence *

1. How soon after you wake up do you smoke your first cigarette?

—After 60 minutes

(0)

—31-60 minutes

(1)

—6-30 minutes

(2)

—Within 5 minutes

(3)

2. Do you find it difficult to refrain from smoking in places where it is forbidden?

—No

(0)

—Yes

(1)

3. Which cigarette would you hate most to give up?

—The first in the morning

(1)

— Any other

(0)

4. How many cigarettes per day do you smoke?

—10 or less

(0)

—11-20

(1)

—21-30

(2)

— 31 or more

(3)

5. Do you smoke more frequently during the first hours after awakening than during the rest of the day?

—No

(0)

—Yes

(1)

6. Do you smoke even if you are so ill that you are in bed most of the day?

—No

(0)

—Yes

(1)

0–2 Very low dependence
3–4 Low dependence
5 Medium dependence
6–7 High dependence
8–10 Very high dependence

[Scores under 5: "Your level of nicotine dependence is still low. You should act now before your level of dependence increases. "]

[Score of 5: "Your level of nicotine dependence is moderate. If you don't quit soon, your level of dependence on nicotine will increase until you may be seriously addicted."]

[Score over 7: "Your level of dependence is high. You aren't in control of your smoking—-it is in control of you!"]

The U.K. Guardian's scoring assessment

Which patch to use:

—**2 points** = light nicotine dependence. Start with the 7 mg nicotine patch.

—**3 or 4 points** = moderate nicotine dependence. Start with the 14 mg nicotine patch.

—**5 or 6 points** = heavy nicotine dependence. Start with the 21 mg nicotine patch.

Friday, February 6, 2009

http://addiction-dirkh.blogspot.com/2009/02/patch-and-how-to-use-it.html

Heatherton TF, Kozlowski LT, Frecker RC, Fagerstrom KO. The Fagerstrom Test for Nicotine Dependence: A revision of the Fagerstrom Tolerance Questionnaire. *British Journal of Addictions.* 86:1119-27. 1991.

Drug Addiction Goes Untreated in Prison

Only 20% of addicted inmates get rehab.

Among the many ironies of the American War on Drugs, the situation of drug abusers in prison ranks high on the list. Despite decades of research showing that drug treatment can be effective, the federal government has failed to offer it consistently, on demand, for prisoners who need rehabilitation. The National Institute on Drug Abuse (NIDA) estimates that only one-fifth of inmates needing formal treatment are able to get it.

Why aren't imprisoned drug addicts getting treatment, instead of ready access to a continuing supply of whatever they are addicted to? **"Addiction is a stigmatized disease that the criminal justice system often fails to view as a medical condition,"** says the report's lead author, Dr. Redonna K. Chandler, chief of NIDA's Services Research Branch. "As a consequence, its treatment is not as available as it is for other medical conditions."

The report, published in the *Journal of the American Medical Association* (JAMA) found that roughly half of all prisoners suffer some degree of drug dependency. "Treating drug abusing offenders improves public health and safety," asserts co-author and NIDA director Dr. Nora D. Volkow, citing increased risk of infectious diseases like HIV and hepatitis C among addicts. **"Providing drug**

abusers with treatment also makes it less likely that these abusers will return to the criminal justice system."

While the high cost of treatment is often cited as a reason for its general absence from the prison infrastructure, Chandler says the cost benefits of treating drug-involved offenders is obvious: "A dollar spent on drug courts saves about $4 in avoided costs of incarceration and health care; and prison-based treatment saves between $2 and $6."

Adds Volkow: "Viewing addiction as a disease does not remove the responsibility of the individual. It highlights the responsibility of the addicted person to get drug treatment and society's responsibility to make treatment available."

Tuesday, January 20, 2009

http://addiction-dirkh.blogspot.com/2009/01/drug-addiction-goes-untreated-in-prison.html

4) Interviews and Book Reviews

(Creative Commons)

An Interview with Pharmacologist David Kroll

On synthetic marijuana, organic medicines, and drugs of the future.

Herewith, a 5-question interview with pharmacologist David Kroll, Ph.D., former Professor and Chair of Pharmaceutical Science at North Carolina Central University in Durham, and a well-known blogger in the online science community.

A cancer pharmacologist whose field is natural products—he has been involved in a project to explore the potential anticancer action of chemicals found in milk thistle and various sorts of fungi—Dr. Kroll received his Ph.D. from the University of Florida, and completed his postdoctoral fellowship in Medical Oncology and Molecular Endocrinology at the University of Colorado School of Medicine. He went on to spend the first nine years of his independent research and teaching career at the University of Colorado School of Pharmacy, where he taught all aspects of pharmacology, from central nervous system-active drugs, to anticancer and antiviral medications. He has also worked as a research pharmacologist for the Research Triangle Institute, and for SmithKline and French Laboratories. He's responsible for Terra Sigillata—a natural products pharmacology and chemistry blog—and Take As Directed, his personal blog. He is also co-author of *Breast Cancer Recurrence and Advanced Disease: Comprehensive Expert Guidance*.

1. *You've been writing about the new synthetic marijuana products on your blog, Terra Sigillata, since they first leaked into the drug underground. Can you briefly explain the origin of these "fake" cannabis chemicals, and the work done by the Huffman lab?*

Every area of CNS pharmacology has chemists who try to figure out the smallest possible chemical structure that can have a biological effect. In fact, this is a longstanding practice of any area of pharmacology. Huffman was an excellent chemist who in the 1990s was trying to figure out the most important part of the active component of marijuana that might have psychotropic effects. These compounds made by him and his students, surprisingly simple ones, I prefer to call cannabimimetics since they mimic the effect of the more complex cannabinoids in marijuana. These basic chemistry and pharmacology studies are what ultimately lead to new drugs in every field - a facet of chemistry called "structure-activity relationships" or SAR.

But since they are simple, they are relatively easy to make - some of Huffman's work at Clemson was actually done by undergraduate chemistry majors. So, it was no surprise that they would be picked up by clandestine drug marketers, even though cannabis (UK) and marijuana (US) are freely available. **The attraction to users was, until recently, that Huffman compounds (prefixed with "JWH-" for his initials) could not be detected in urine by routine drug testing. Hence, incense products containing these compounds have been called "probationer's weed."**

2. *In a guest blog post for Scientific American titled "Drugs from the Crucible of Nature," you remind us that several hundred common drugs are modified natural products. What stands in the way of discovering, isolating, and testing more of these plant drugs?*

Fully 25% of all pharmaceuticals can trace their roots to natural products: chemicals made by plants, bacteria, fungi, and marine creatures that possess biological effects in mammals. **The first**

ones we recognized as humans were those which altered our perception of reality or our ability to adapt to the strenuous, pre-modern life: hallucinogens for religious purposes and stimulants to support physical activity and suppress hunger. Over time, we found other drugs that treated pain (opiates), heart failure or "dropsy" (digitalis), or cancerous lesions (podophyllin from the Penobscot Native Americans).

We know today that natural products have much greater chemical diversity than drugs made by man and are useful additions to the study of new drug targets. However, naturally-occurring drugs sometimes have major drawbacks: they are difficult to make in the laboratory or require large amounts of their natural source to be commercially viable, they can have undesired effects that may not be apparent from traditional uses, or they require chemical modifications to be safer, more resistant to metabolism, and to become patentable intellectual property.

Over the last 10-15 years, the short-term, investor- and market-driven view of pharmaceutical companies has led the big firms to eliminate their natural product research programs. **Today, much of the discovery of naturally occurring drugs has been left to academic researchers and small companies where many former pharma researchers reside.** Once we get compounds that may be viewed as "druggable" by the pharmaceutical industry or the National Cancer Institute (in the US), they can then move to clinical trials.

3. *Psychoactive plant drugs like the poppy played a major role in the development of modern pharmacology and neurology. One school of thought says that psychoactive drugs are overprescribed, addictive, and ineffective panaceas. The other side views such drugs as targeted, effective, and increasingly sophisticated treatments for diseases once thought to be untreatable. Have we become a nation of crazed pill heads, or is this simply pharmaceutical medicine on the march?*

I have a middle-of-the-road view on this topic. As you know (and my blog readers will know) my father suffered from alcoholism that was comorbid with clinical depression. **Real, biochemically-based depression has been undertreated in Western societies, in part due to the stigma that admitting mental disorders is somehow viewed as compromising one's intellect.** Nothing could be farther from the truth, of course. Some of the most brilliant and creative minds in all fields have suffered from depression, mania, and, sadly, ended their lives early by suicide.

So, drugs certainly have their place for those unfairly dealt a hand of bad brain biochemistry. We should not view this as any worse than getting the bad genes for hypertension or diabetes. The problem seems to be those with mild-to-moderate psychiatric disorders, many of which can be managed without drugs but that require personal effort in the form of psychotherapy, cognitive behavioral therapy, or other flavors of hard, personal work. As Americans, what do we want? The hard work or the pill? If we want to lose weight, do we want exercise, caloric restriction, or a pill? Hence, we are the ones who are complicit with pharmaceutical companies. We want the pill rather than the hard work and the companies supply that demand. **Anyone who doesn't realize that we as a society facilitate what we demonize in pharmaceutical companies is just simply in denial.**

4. *It's increasingly obvious that our legal and cultural approaches to addictive drugs have not been successful. What's your take on the drug war, and on the problematic distinction between "legal" and "illegal" drugs of abuse?*

My primary research field is cancer drugs, but my teaching brings me into the realm of drugs of abuse, simply because so many of those drugs are naturally-occurring. So, my views must be taken in that perspective. In the US, I think that it is morally difficult to justify the legality of addictive drugs like alcohol and tobacco while restricting other psychoactive compounds. I do not advocate for other drugs to be used recreationally. I just feel that US laws need to be consistent. Our experiment with criminalizing alcohol was an abysmal failure that fostered organized crime. Our continued experiment with criminalizing other drugs has been equally a failure. However, I am very much against a libertarian argument that society should be free to determine what they want because, frankly, many drugs impair one's decision-making ability.

But I like your question: many drugs declared illegal for recreational use are among the most useful therapeutics for pain, especially the pain associated with surgery and cancer. **My greater humanistic concern is that our society's zero tolerance approach to drugs that "could" be illegal is that people who need them for their desired effect often go without.** Undermanagement of pain is the major casualty of the war on drugs. No, let me fix that. People who suffer unnecessarily from pain when useful drugs could be used are the major casualties of the war on drugs.

5. *What's going on in pharmaceutical research these days that has you excited?*

When I was graduating with my toxicology degree in 1985 from the Philadelphia College of Pharmacy and Science, I asked my chairman Dr. Gary Lage where I should expect new drugs to come from. His words of wisdom were that I should pay close attention— not to drug companies, but rather to major advances in physiology. Learning that the kidney played a role in red blood cell count led to the use of erythropoeitin for anemia caused by renal failure and chemotherapy.

Today, I see major drug targets in the epigenome— the part of genetics that is affected by environmental influences. We are all stuck with the static part of our inherited

DNA—the exact base sequences and their polymorphisms and mutations. However, we're learning that those things can be modified by diet, environmental exposures, and, yes, drugs. The epigenome is a broad target for a multitude of diseases, never more complicated but never more promising.

Thursday, September 22, 2011

http://addiction-dirkh.blogspot.com/2011/09/
interview-with-pharmacologist-david.html

The Hidden Story of How Big Tobacco Invented Freebasing

Review of The Golden Holocaust: Origins of the Cigarette Catastrophe and the Case for Abolition.

It's easy to think of cigarettes, and the machinations of the tobacco industry, as "old news." But in his revealing 737-page book, The Golden Holocaust, based on 70 million pages of documents from the tobacco industry, Stanford professor Robert N. Proctor demonstrates otherwise. He demonstrates how Big Tobacco invented freebasing. He shows how they colluded in misleading the public about "safe" alternatives like filters, "low-tar," and "ultra-lights." We discover in Lorillard's archives an explanation of menthol's appeal to African Americans: It is all part of a desire by "negroes" to mask a "genetic body odor." Radioactive isotopes were isolated in cigarette smoke, and evidence of the find was published, as early as 1953. He reveals that the secret ingredient in Kent's "micronite filter" was asbestos. And he charges that the "corruption of science" lies behind the industry's drive to continue its deadly trade. "Collaboration with the tobacco industry," writes Proctor, "is one of the most deadly abuses of scholarly integrity in modern history."

Half of all cigarette smokers will die from smoking—about a billion people this century, if present trends continue. In the U.S., this translates into roughly two jumbo jets crashing, killing everyone onboard, once daily. Cigarettes kill more people than bullets. The world smokes 6 *trillion* of them each year. (The Chinese alone account for about 2 trillion). Some people believe that tobacco represents a problem (more or less) solved, at least in the developed West.

All of this represents a continuing triumph for the tobacco industry. The aiders and abettors of tobacco love to portray the tobacco story as "old news." **But as Stanford Professor Robert M. Proctor writes in** *The Golden Holocaust,* **his exhaustive history of tobacco science and industry: "Global warming denialists cut their teeth on tobacco tactics, fighting science with science, creating doubt, fostering ignorance."**

Checking in at 737 pages, *The Golden Holocaust* is nobody's idea of a light read, and at times its organization seems clear only to the author. But what a treasure trove of buried facts and misleading science Proctor has uncovered, thanks to more than 70 million pages of industry documents now online (http://legacy.library.ucsf. edu) as part of the Master Settlement Agreement of 1998. Once the material was finally digitized and available online, scholars like Proctor could employ full-text optical character recognition for detailed searchability. Ironically, this surreal blizzard of documentation was meant to obscure meaningful facts, not make them readily available, but tobacco executives seem not to have factored in digital technology when they turned over the material.

The single most important technological breakthrough in the history of the modern cigarette was flue-curing, which lowers the pH of tobacco smoke enough to make it inhalable. The reason few people inhale cigars, and very few used to inhale cigarettes, is that without some help, burning tobacco has a pH too high for comfortable inhalation. It makes you cough. But flue-curing lowered pH levels, allowing for a "milder," less alkaline smoke that even women and children could tolerate.

World War I legitimized cigarettes in a major way. Per capita consumption in the U.S. almost tripled from 1914 to 1919, which

Proctor considers "one of the most rapid increases in smoking ever recorded." After World War II, the Marshall Plan shipped a staggering $1 billion worth of tobacco and other "food-related items." (The U.S. Senator who blustered the loudest for big postwar tobacco shipments to Europe was A. Willis Robertson of Virginia, the father of televangelist Pat Robertson.)

The military, as we know, has historically been gung-ho on cigarettes. **And Proctor claims that "the front shirt pocket that now adorns the dress of virtually every American male, for example, was born from an effort to make a place to park your cigarette pack."** In addition, cigarette makers spent a great deal of time and effort convincing automakers and airline manufacturers to put ashtrays into the cars and planes they sold. Ashtrays were built into seats in movie theaters, barbershops, and lecture halls. There was even an ashtray built into the U.S. military's anti-Soviet SAGE computer in the 50s.

In the early 50s, research by Ernest Wynder in the U.S. and Angel Roffo in Argentina produced the first strong evidence that tobacco tars caused cancer in mice. Roffo in particular seemed convinced that tobacco caused lung cancer, that it was the tar rather than the nicotine, and that the main culprits were the aromatic hydrocarbons such as benzpyrene. **Curiously enough, it was influential members of Germany's Third Reich in the 40s who first took the possibility of a link seriously.** Hans Reiter, a powerful figure in public health in Germany, said in a 1941 speech that smoking had been linked to human lung cancers through "painstaking observations of individual cases."

In the December 1953 issue of *Cancer Research,* Wynder, et al. published a paper demonstrating that "tars extracted from tobacco smoke could induce cancers when painted on the skins of mice." As it turns out, the tobacco industry already knew it. Executives had funded their own research, while keeping a close eye on outside academic studies, and had been doing so since at least the 30s. **In fact, French doctors had been referring to cancers des fumeurs, or smokers' cancers, since the mid-1800s.** All of which knocks the first leg out from under the tobacco industry's classic position: We didn't know any stuff about cancer hazards until well into the 1950s.

Only weeks after the Wynder paper was published, tobacco execs went into full conspiracy mode during a series of meetings at the Plaza Hotel in New York, "where the denialist campaign was set in motion." American Tobacco Company President Paul Hahn issued a press release that came to be known as the "Frank Statement" of 1954. Proctor calls it the "magna carta of the American's industry's conspiracy to deny any evidence of tobacco harms." **How, Proctor asks, did science get shackled to the odious enterprise of exonerating cigarettes?** The secret was not so much in out-right suppression of science, though there was plenty of that: In one memorable action known as the "Mouse House Massacre," R.J. Reynolds abruptly shut down their internal animal research lab and laid off 26 scientists overnight, after the researchers began obtaining unwelcome results about tobacco smoke. But the true genius of the industry "was rather in using even 'good' science, narrowly defined, as a *distraction*, something to hold up to say, in effect: See how responsible we are?"

Entities like the Council for Tobacco Research engaged in decoy research of this kind. As one tobacco company admitted, "Research must go on and on."

A good deal of the industry's research in the 50s and 60s was in fact geared toward reverse engineering competitors' successes. Consider Marlboro. Every cigarette manufacturer want to know: How did they do it? What was the secret to Marlboro's success?

As it turns out, they did it by increasing nicotine's kick. And they accomplished that, in essence, by means of freebasing, a process invented by the cigarette industry. **Adding ammonia or some other alkaline compound transforms a molecule of nicotine from its bound salt version to its "free" base, which volatilizes much more easily, providing low-pH smoke easily absorbed by body tissue.** And there you have the secret: "The freebasing of cocaine hydrochloride into 'crack' is based on a similar chemistry: the cocaine alkaloid is far more potent in its free base form than as a salt, so bicarbonate is used to transform cocaine hydrochloride into chemically pure crack cocaine." Once other cigarette makers figured out the formula, they too began experimenting with the advantages of an "enhanced alkaline environment."

Wednesday, May 23, 2012

http://addiction-dirkh.blogspot.com/2012/05/hidden-story-of-how-big-tobacco.html

Review: Memoirs of an Addicted Brain

"I'm a drug addict turned neuroscientist."

What's it like to swallow 400 milligrams of dextromethorphan hydrobromide, better known as Romilar cough syrup? "Flashes of perception go by like clumps of scenery on either side, while you float along with the slow, irresistible momentum of a dream." Marc Lewis, a former addict, now a practicing neuroscientist, further muses: **"But what was Romilar? It sounded like an ancient kingdom. Would this dark elixir take me to some faraway place? Would it take me into another land? Would it be hard to come back?"**

In *Memoirs of an Addicted Brain: A Neuroscientist Examines his Former Life on Drugs*, Dr. Marc Lewis follows his description of his gateway Romilar drug experience with the neurological basics of the matter: "The problem is that the NMDA receptors in my brain are now clogged with dextromethorphan molecules! The glutamate isn't getting through. The receptor neurons aren't firing, or they're not firing fast enough.... Drugs like DM, ketamine, PCP, angel dust, and those most damaging of substances, glue and gasoline, are called dissociatives, because they do exactly what drugs are supposed to do: they dissociate feeling from reality, meaning from sense—and that's *all* they do."

Speaking of the self-reinforcing cycle "through which calamities of the mind arise from vulnerabilities of the brain," Lewis argues that dissociatives only produce an absence. As a friend of his puts it with regard to another popular dissociative, "Nitrous oxide doesn't give you consciousness. It takes it away." And then, the friend adds: "Just bonk yourself on the head with a baseball bat if you want to lose consciousness."

Lewis ultimately turns to opioids. "The emotional circuitry of the ventral striatum seems to derive its power from an intimate discourse between opioid *liking* and dopamine wanting." In the end, this partnership does more than produce pleasure. **It also, Lewis points out, "gets us to work for things." And by doing that, addictive drugs demonstrate "the fundamental chemistry of *learning* which really means learning what feels good and how to get more of it. Yet there's a downside: the slippery slope, the repetition compulsion, that constitutes addiction.** In other words, addiction may be a form of learning gone bad. For me, this neurochemical sleight of hand promises much more pain than pleasure in the years to come."

Lewis does a good job of capturing the feeling of existential despair brought on by uncontrolled addiction: "Contemptible. That's what I was. Unbelievably stupid, unbelievably irresponsible: selfish, selfish, selfish! But that wasn't quite it. What described me, what this inner voice accused me of, wasn't exactly selfish, not exactly weak, but some meridian of self-blame that included both, and also, dirty, disgusting... maybe just BAD."

How did heroin feel? "I feel relief from that pervasive hiss of wrongness. Every emotional wound, every bruise, every ache in my psyche, the background noise of angst itself, is soaked with a balm of unbelievable potency. There is a ringing stillness. The sense of impending harm, of danger, of attack, both from within and without, is washed away."

And Lewis provides a memorable summation of the reward system, as dopamine streams from the ventral tegmental area to its targets, "the ventral striatum, where behavior is charged, focused, and released; the orbitofrontal cortex, where it infuses cells devoted to the *value* of this drug; and the amygdala, whose synapses provide a meeting place for the two most important components of associative memory, imagery and emotion." **In fact, "dopamine-powered desperation can change the brain forever, because its message of *intense wanting* narrows the field of synaptic change, focusing it like a powerful microscope on one particular reward. Whether in the service of food or heroin, love or gambling, dopamine forms a rut, a line of footprints in the neural flesh."**

And, of course, Lewis relapses, and eventually ends his addictive years in an amphetamine-induced psychosis, committing serial burglaries to fund his habit. "You'd think that getting busted, put on probation, kicked out of graduate school, and enduring a kind of infamy that was agonizing to experience and difficult to hide—all of that, and the need to start life over again—would be enough to get me to stop. It wasn't."

Not then, anyway. But Lewis has been clean now for 30 years. "Nobody likes an addict," he writes. "Not even other addicts."

If drugs are such feel-good engines, what goes wrong? Something big. "Because when drugs (or booze, sex, or gambling) are nowhere to be found, when the horizon is empty of their promise, the humming motor of the orbitofrontal cortex sputters to a halt. Orbitofrontal cells go dormant and dopamine just stops. Like a religious fundamentalist, the addict's brain has only two stable states: rapture and disinterest. Addictive drugs convert the brain to recognize only one face of God, to thrill to only one suitor." The addict's world narrows. Dopamine becomes "specialized, stilted, inaccessible through the ordinary pleasures and pursuits of life, but gushing suddenly when anything associated with the drug comes into awareness.... I wish this were just an exercise in biological reductionism, or neuro-scientific chauvinism, but it's not. It's the way things really work."

Friday, May 4, 2012

http://addiction-dirkh.blogspot.com/2012/05/review-memoirs-of-addicted-brain.html

Ivan Oransky on the Disease Model at TEDMED

What we think about when we think about "disease."

It's a safe bet that the number of M.D.s who have made a mid-career switch to journalism is rather small. And when Dr. Ivan Oransky did it, he didn't go in for half measures. The former online editor of *Scientific American*, and the former deputy editor of *The Scientist*, Oransky now serves as Executive Editor of *Reuters Health*. He teaches medical journalism at New York University, where he also holds an appointment as clinical assistant professor of medicine—while maintaining three, yes three, separate blogs. He is well known for two innovative blogs known as Retraction Watch and Embargo Watch. And he recently kicked off a personal blog, the Oransky Journal.

So clearly, he's a very lazy man. Nonetheless, he found time to give a very popular talk on the shortcomings of the disease model of medicine at last week's TEDMED conference in Washington, D.C. And he found additional time to grant me an interview afterwards, with some interesting thoughts on how the mania for medicalization could affect addiction treatment.

Speaking at the Kennedy Center for the Performing Arts, Oransky compared patients in the nation's current medical system to baseball coach Billy Beane, a once-promising player who washed out in the minors and was recently portrayed by Brad Pitt in the movie Moneyball. **"Our medical system is just as bad at predicting what's happening to patients as baseball scouts were at predicting what would happen to Billy Beane,"** **Oransky told the audience of 1,500.**

"Every day, thousands of people across the country are diagnosed with pre-conditions," he said. "We hear about pre-hypertension, we hear about pre-dementia and pre-anxiety. We also refer to sub-clinical conditions, like sub-clinical hardening of the arteries. One of my favorites is called sub-clinical acne. If you look up their website as I did, you'll see that they say this is the easiest acne to treat. You don't have any pustules or inflammation—you don't actually have acne. I have a name for preconditions—I call them preposterous."

Every year, according to Oransky, "we are spending more than two trillion dollars on health care," and yet more than 100,000 people a year are dying from complications of the treatments they're getting, rather than from the conditions that are being treated. And most patient advocacy groups eventually learn to "expand the number of people who are eligible for a given treatment" for fundraising purposes, he said.

As evidence of this trend toward medicalization, Oransky pointed to the novel notion of a "previvor." According to FORCE, the cancer research advocacy group that coined the term: "A previvor is a survivor of a predisposition to cancer." The term is used to describe someone who, for example, has a genetic risk for breast cancer, but has not been diagnosed with the disease. "Previvor was coined in 2000 after a challenge from a community member who said she 'needed a label,'" according to the group's web site.

We are all previvors of some disorder, Oransky argues. In the spirit of giving everyone a precondition, Oransky coined the term "pre-death." **What is pre-death? "Every single one of you** has it," Oransky told the audience, "because you have the risk factor for it, which is being alive."

Using his favorite metaphor—baseball—Oransky explained the secret of Billy Beane's revolutionary success as a coach: "The secret wasn't to swing at every pitch, like the sluggers do. You had to find the guys who liked to walk, because getting on base by a walk is just as good. And in our health care system, we need to figure out, 'is that really a good pitch, or do we need to let it go by, and not swing at everything?' We all need to keep in mind that in medicine, sometimes less is more."

After his talk, I asked Oransky how the theme of medicalization might apply to the disease of addiction. Medicalization, he said, is a matter of "taking advantage of people, manipulating them so they can't make informed decisions." **In the case of addiction treatment, Oransky pointed to the "proliferation of ads for treatment in beautiful places. It's all selling and self-diagnosis. They're selling you on the fact that you need to be treated."** He also pointedly referred to the practice of "medical astro-turfing," where a supposedly grass roots effort by patients or advocates is "usurped by interest group pressure." Sometimes that usurpation is patently obvious, is in the case of many advocacy groups set in motion and funded by pharmaceutical companies or the liquor industry.

Sometimes, of course, you do need to be treated. **And Oransky notes that in health areas such as addiction and mental illness—disorders where social stigma remains high, compared to, say, a blood infection—there are "fewer pressures to medicalize."** And possibly, too few pressures to medicalize. "There's no quick and easy test, no MRI where you can point to the place in the brain that lights up and say, 'you are an alcoholic.'" The science of addiction, which has been moving by fits and starts into the medical mainstream, has a long way to go, compared with many other disease categories. And it has left a gap through which medical workers and treatment staff can march, chanting, "I have a system," Oransky says.

Perhaps, then, the study of addiction to alcohol and other drugs requires both more medicalization of the research kind, and less of the "precondition" or "sub-clinical" kind. As for the second kind, Oransky believes we are already medicalizing binge drinking in a counterproductive way. **In addition, "there are always attempts to widen the market. Look at how obesity has been made to overlap with addiction."** As for medications being used to combat craving among addicts in treatment, Oransky noted the tendency to "repurpose" drugs on the basis of soft data. "They took wellbutrin, an antidepressant that didn't work very well, and offered it for smoking cessation. So I would want to see data that is really robust" before treating addicts with such medications.

On the other hand, Oransky noted, "We don't have to worry about malaria, we don't need to medicalize tuberculosis. **But do diseases that have a strong stigma, like addiction, actually *benefit* from medicalization? If we find out that they do, than we should do it."**

There's something else Oransky believes is overdue for true medicalization: "The social determinants of health care—poverty, the way we build our suburban environments. Concentrate on stuff that we know kills people. Medicalize that."

In the end, he said, "we need to use marketing strategies to effectively get treatment to the people who need it, not to the people who don't."

Sunday, April 15, 2012

http://addiction-dirkh.blogspot.com/2012/04/
ivan-oransky-on-disease-model-at-tedmed.html

Interview with Cognitive Neuropsychologist Keith Laws

LSD, E, CBT, and "Mind-Pops."

Dr. Keith Laws, professor of cognitive neuropsychology and head of research in the School of Psychology at the University of Hertfordshire, UK, holds a Ph.D. from the Department of Experimental Psychology at the University of Cambridge, and is the author of *Category-Specificity: Evidence for Modularity of Mind*. He has written extensively on cognitive deficits resulting from certain types of neurological injury, and has won several awards for his research on cognitive functioning in schizophrenia. He also maintains an active interest in the challenges of functional brain imaging. Professor Laws is frequently quoted in the British media, and is the author of more than 100 peer-reviewed articles. He is a Chartered Psychologist and an Associate Fellow of the British Psychological Society. And recently, Professor Laws became a blogger, launching the LawsNeuroBlog. He maintains a web homepage, and is virtually unbeatable in the category of obscure British rock trivia.

1. LSD is back in the news, with a rehash of several old studies on acid and alcoholism. A lot of people would like to revive research interest in LSD, MDMA, magic mushrooms, and other psychedelics.What's your view?

Keith Laws: Yes, "re-hash" is an appropriate phrase—we are witnessing a rebranding of "counter-culture" as "over-the-counter-culture."The history of LSD research is frequently retold as if grand therapeutic advances were halted because hostile governments criminalised LSD. The bottom-line, however, is that most studies of the 50s and 60s produced little worthy of further scientific pursuit. The recent meta-analysis of 60s studies examining whether LSD reduces "alcohol misuse" is a case in point.

That meta-analysis consisted of 6 trials—none of which produced a significant effect, but their total pooled effect suggested some impact on alcohol misuse. In my recent post on this study, I highlighted a series of points, including: how it is likely that further negative studies have been gathering dust in the file drawers of researchers over the years; how some samples consisted of people with serious comorbid mental health and neurological problems (schizophrenia, epilepsy, organic brain disorder, low IQ); and crucially, how the authors made the totally unfounded assumption that anyone dropping-out of the studies had relapsed into drinking. This had a large and disproportionate impact on the control samples in those studies—as many more dropped out from control groups. **Combined with the lack of significant effects in any one study, doubts exist about relying on these data as a justification for starting large-scale trials of LSD for alcoholism. We should certainly skeptically regard statements by some, such as Professor David Nutt, that LSD is "as good as anything we've got for treating alcoholism."**

2. Tell us about your research interest in the effect of Ecstasy (MDMA) on memory.

Keith Laws: First, I think its crucial not to confuse E and MDMA. Studies of MDMA in humans are few, and mostly examine acute effects via self-report. The vast majority of studies though, including our work, examine the residual effects of street-E in abstinent users i.e. taking largely unknown compounds mixed with varying degrees of MDMA. For me, the real public health issue relates to street-E since most people outside of the lab rarely get to consume pure MDMA.

In 2007 we meta-analysed 26 studies that had examined memory on standardized tests in over 600 ecstasy users and 600 non-users and found significant long and short-term verbal memory impairments in 75% of users. Intriguingly, E was unrelated to visual memory problems; however those who also smoked cannabis did display significant visual memory impairment. A key finding of ours was that the lifetime number of E tablets consumed was unrelated to the degree of memory impairment. This led to a host of misrepresentations in the media and amongst E users who saw it as license to take as many Es as they want. I view this finding, however in a much starker light—taking E is akin to playing Russian Roulette with your memory. **Some may tolerate 100s or even 1000s of E tablets, but for others far fewer may lead to memory problems—we can predict that 3 in 4 users will develop memory problems, but not which 3 or after how many tablets.** Of course, ecstasy (like Cannabis) is often advocated as a safe-ish drug because it rarely kills. Indeed, metrics of drug harm developed in the UK emphasise physical and social harm, but fail to explicitly acknowledge the cognitive problems associated with E and other recreational drugs. Given that as many as 500,000 young people in the UK use E each week and 75% are affected, then that's 375,000 young people developing significant verbal memory problems!

3.You're not convinced by the findings of a recent study of magic mushrooms, where the researchers documented an overall decrease in brain activity.What else could account for this effect?

Keith Laws: Well, the surprising thing about the Carhart-Harris et. al. psilocybin study was the general pattern of brain deactivation, which contrasts with the findings of activation in others such as Vollenweider and colleagues in Switzerland who find increased activation. The decreased activation especially in the medial prefrontal cortex (mPFC) and the posterior cingulate cortex (PCC) were curious and reminded me of the similar deactivation in these areas linked both to anxiety and to the anticipation of unpleasant events. **It occurred to me that the prospect of tripping in a scanner may be quite anxiety provoking, and several features of the study led to me to think this may have been the case.** First the order of testing was always the same - participants received the placebo scan always before the psilocybin scan and so, could always anticipate the trip— potentially heightening anxious anticipation in that condition. Second, Carhart-Harris et. al. measured "anxiety" and "fear of losing one's mind" and both multiplied many fold in the psilocybin condition. Interestingly and subsequently, Vollenweider and colleagues pooled date from 23 studies and found that experimental settings involving scanning most strongly predicted unpleasant and/or anxious reactions to psilocybin - converging directly on my suspicion. Although nobody would deny that hallucinogens such as psilocybin impact brain function - the question is which parts reflect the "trip" and which parts reflect "anxiety about the trip"?

4.You have also looked at the matter of using cognitive behavioral therapy for various kinds of mental disorders. How does CBT measure up, in your opinion? Is it useful for addiction?

Keith Laws: Yes, unlike any other country, the UK endorses using CBT to treat psychotic symptoms and to prevent relapse in schizophrenia. Indeed, "NICE" (the National Institute of Clinical Excellence), which decide which treatments are made available to UK patients, suggest that we offer CBT to "all people with schizophrenia". Anyway, we meta-analysed the data for whether CBT reduces symptomatology or prevents relapse and came to the conclusion that the evidence supports neither. Crucially, CBT only appeared to "work" when the therapists were not blind at outcome assessment i.e. they knew to which group the patient was assigned (CBT or control)! The irony is that CBT therapists sing the mantra of evidence-based practice!

In terms of the use of CBT in people with substance abuse problems, it produces a small impact on abstinence with opiates, stimulants and cocaine, but has little or impact on alcohol use; and as one might expect, these effects disappear across time. Some evidence also suggests that women respond better to CBT than men. **Perhaps the most intriguing finding in this area is that CBT has had much greater success in reducing cannabis use, with up to 80% showing significant reduction in use.**

5.What else have you been investigating recently? What are you excited about?

Keith Laws: Over the past 3 years or so I have been doing more work with individuals suffering from the obsessive compulsive syndrome of disorders i.e. OCD, Body Dysmorphic Disorder, Trichotillomania, Schizo-Obsessive disorder, Tourette's, and Perfectionism. Our work is looking at phenotypes that might be expressed through this range of disorders and in their first-degree unaffected relatives.

Other things we are working on include what we call "Mind-Pops"—those little thoughts, words, images, or tunes that suddenly pop into your mind at unexpected times and are totally unrelated to your current activity— described long ago by novelists such as Marcel Proust and Vladimir Nabokov. We have just published a paper showing that verbal hallucinations, the core symptom of schizophrenia, may be related to the mind-pop phenomenon that almost everybody experiences, but just manifests itself in a different way.

Sunday, April 1, 2012

http://addiction-dirkh.blogspot.com/2012/04/interview-with-cognitive.html

Steve Earle and the Ghost of Hank Williams

Book Review: *I'll Never Get Out of This World Alive.*

Musician Steve Earle made a solo name for himself with *Guitar Town* and *Copperhead Road* after playing in legendary country and bluegrass bands as a young prodigy. He was nominated for a Grammy, his reputations soared, he added rock and roll to his range—until 1991, when Earle put out the aptly named live album, *Shut Up and Die Like An Aviator*. **Shortly thereafter, he was dropped by his record label for long-standing drug problems, and landed in prison with a heavy sentence for possession of heroin.** He completed rehab successfully, earned his parole in 1994, and has gone on since then to make several highly successful albums, guest star in the TV series *The Wire*, and write music for the New Orleans-based series *Treme*.

And now he has written a novel called *I'll Never Get out of This World Alive,* set mostly in San Antonio, with a main character who is an aging doctor and a heroin addict. Doc's specialty is quick but relatively safe and sterile backroom abortions, commonly performed on illegal immigrants. His license to practice long ago taken away, Doc takes in enough to make his daily pilgrimage to the parking lot where his longtime dealer works the streets. **The book's title is taken from the name of a Hank Williams song, which is appropriate, because whether or not you enjoy this novel**

may depend upon your reaction to Hank's ghost hanging around the main character, begging for a drink and some attention. Things get even stranger when a young Mexican girl, Graciela, falls under the doctor's care, and begins to exhibit signs of stigmata and the power to heal drug addicts. **Rather than choosing to tell his tale straightforwardly, Earle is working more in the tradition of Latin American magical realism.** This is no *One Hundred Years of Solitude*, but a lot hangs on belief, and the power of unseen forces to organize events in unforeseen ways.

Earle has a fun, quick touch with character description and the telling anecdote, explaining, for example, that local narcotic detective Hugo Ackerman "rarely hurried even when attempting to catch a fleeing offender. He had worked narcotics for over a decade, and in his experience neither the junkies nor the pushers were going far. He caught up with everybody eventually."

Set in 1963, the book carries us through the Kennedy assassination and other cultural events as background. And we get a nice, deft description of what starts the doctor down the road toward smackdom: "Then in the first year of his residency he befriended a crazy old pathologist who worked the midnight shift in the county morgue, and it was he who introduced Doc to the miracle of morphine. From that very first shot it was as if he'd discovered the one vital ingredient that God had left out when He'd send Doc kicking and screaming into the cold, cruel world."

I won't say that Mr. Earle should give up his day job on the basis of this outing, but I do think that critics who have dismissed his efforts have overlooked some of what the author is attempting to say about addiction, and about recovery—that recovery involves all kinds of intangibles like faith, hope and charity, and that these attributes can present themselves in myriad disguises. (And a lot of critics got it: Michael Ondaatje wrote that this "subtle and dramatic book is the work of a brilliant songwriter who has moved from song to orchestral ballad with astonishing ease.")

I think this book is, in fact, written very much with addicts in mind. The shade of Hank Williams doesn't dog Doc everywhere just because Steve Earle is a huge fan. **Hank Williams was also a vicious, go-to-hell alcoholic and drug addict who could not make the turnaround Steve Earle has made, and therefore could not even get out of his twenties alive, let alone this world.** Earle has Doc stand in for him when it comes to lessons learned: "Doc was immediately sucked in by the big lie that all junkies want to believe in spite of daily evidence to the contrary, that this shot was going to be like that first shot all those years ago. He tied off, found the money vein in the back of his arm, well rested now because he had always reserved that one for the big shots, the teeth rattlers, and it stood at attention like a soldier on payday."

I won't give out any spoilers here, as the miraculous Graciela bleeds from her wounds and lays hands on dying addicts to save them. It's the stuff of, well, fiction—but fiction informed by the author's firsthand voyage into heroin bondage. Steve Earle is living proof of the overarching theme of his book: redemption in its many guises.

Monday, May 30, 2011

http://addiction-dirkh.blogspot.com/2011/05/steve-earle-and-ghost-of-hank-williams.html

An Interview with
Neuroscientist Jon Simons

Brain scans, iPhone love, and state-dependent memory.

Brain scans have put cognitive neuroscience on the map. They have become a key part of addiction studies as well. In fact, brain scans have put neuroscience on the front page, due to the controversies they have engendered. Cognitive neuroscientist Jon Simons, a lecturer in the Department of Experimental Psychology at the University of Cambridge, UK, and principal investigator at the University's Memory Laboratory, is attempting to expand our understanding of the specific regions of the brain involved in human memory. His research involves functional neuroimaging of healthy volunteers and examining the effects of neurological and psychiatric disorders, and normal aging, on memory abilities.

Dr. Simons obtained his PhD at the MRC Cognition and Brain Sciences Unit in Cambridge, and from there moved to a post-doctoral position at Harvard University. He returned to the UK and took up a research fellowship at University College London before returning to Cambridge. He was recently senior author on a thought-provoking paper published in the *Journal of Neuroscience* about a brain structure variation that might explain why some people in the general population are better than others at distinguishing real events from those they imagined or were told about.

1. *PET and fMRI scans have stirred up a good deal of debate and heated argument lately. While brain scans have been used to extend our understanding of crucial functions like memory and reward, they've also been used to "prove" that we're addicted to our iPhones. Some scientists put almost no faith in them at all. What's going on?*

Neuroimaging methods like fMRI have certainly become quite common in the media over recent years. Unfortunately, not all the media coverage does the kind of job we might wish in explaining the methods and findings and, importantly, the limitations and caveats that need to be considered when interpreting the data. You mention the recent *New York Times* op-ed in which it was claimed that people "literally love their iPhones," on the basis that viewing an iPhone was associated with fMRI activity in a brain region previously linked with "love and compassion." **Unfortunately, the same brain area has also been linked with negative emotions like disgust, as well as many other cognitive functions, seriously undermining the claims in the *New York Times* story.** It may turn out to be true that our feelings about iPhones reflect love, or perhaps more likely a kind of dopamine-driven addiction response, but such simplistic analyses as the one the NYT gave such prominence are unlikely to help with understanding that.

However, I think it's a mistake to confuse the media representation of fMRI research with the field itself. Many researchers design very careful fMRI experiments in which factors of interest are varied while others are controlled, and resulting patterns of brain activity are analysed with statistical caution and interpreted in the light of a broad range of previous findings. This is the kind of work that is moving the field forward, but, like most good science, it is not particularly sexy, and the researchers involved are less keen to make the kinds of extravagant claims that get you into the *New York Times*. **In my view, it's up to all of us—scientists and journalists—to make sure that the public get to hear more**

about the good fMRI work, and less about silly iPhone love stories.

2. Is there a specific role for functional neuroimaging in the diagnosis and treatment of addiction?

This isn't really my area, but I know from talking with colleagues that neuroimaging has certainly contributed to understanding the neurobiology of addiction. For example, a great deal is known about the brain networks and neurotransmitter systems implicated in impulsivity, compulsions, reward processing and other cognitive functions that are relevant to addiction disorders. Such knowledge is obviously very important for informing clinical practice. **Whether neuroimaging can also play a role in diagnosis and treatment is, as far as I can tell, less clear.** Making accurate diagnoses in an individual on the basis of neuroimaging data requires characterisation of the specific patterns of brain activity exhibited by that individual, which is difficult to achieve. Similar problems afflict attempts to assess the success of different treatments. However, as imaging technology develops and statistical methods are refined, it may be that neuroimaging will be able to offer new insights that contribute to effective diagnosis and treatment.

3. Please explain the basics of state-dependent memory as it relates to alcohol, using your famous example about remembering Brad Pitt's or Angelina Jolie's phone number.

Ha! Glad if the example I used has proven memorable. **The basic idea of state-dependent memory is that your recollection of a previous event is likely to be better if you're in the same physiological state as you were when the event occurred.** So, to use alcohol as an example, if you're at a party and happen to drunkenly strike up conversation with Angelina Jolie (or Brad Pitt, if you prefer) and, bowled over by your charm and witty repartee, she tells you her phone number, you may well not remember it when you wake up sober the next morning. However, the evidence from many state-dependent memory studies suggests that you would have a better chance of recalling the number if you got drunk again. **The effect doesn't just apply to alcohol: any physiological state, any emotion we're feeling, in fact any aspect of the context we're in when we try to remember, which was also there when we previously experienced an event, will improve our memory for that event.** This was described as the 'encoding specificity principle' by a great memory researcher, Endel Tulving.

4. Some researchers maintain that mental illness and addiction to drugs and alcohol are not, properly speaking, diseases at all. What's your stance on the continual battles over the "disease model" of addiction and other disorders like depression?

There are both advantages and disadvantages to the "disease model" of cognitive disorders. For some people, it might be helpful to receive a clinical disease diagnosis and, perhaps, an idea of the therapeutic interventions through which they might go about "recovering" from their condition. Among the disadvantages are that labelling people as "addicts", for example, can stigmatise those struggling with dependence and might lead to them avoiding responsibility for changing their addictive behaviour because they see diseases as requiring expert intervention. It's a difficult area, and I can see both sides of the debate.

5. You've done neuroscience at Cambridge in the U.K., and at Harvard in the U.S. Is science conducted differently in the two countries?

My experience was that science in the US at that time (in 2000-2001) was different from in the UK. There seemed to be many more opportunities to get involved in interesting projects and to gain access to advanced technical equipment like fMRI scanners than was the case in the UK then. I also noted a difference in the willingness of people who were experts in techniques like fMRI, or in research involving patients with rare brain lesions, to share their expertise and resources in a collaborative way. Fortunately, I've found since I've been back in the UK a similarly friendly and collaborative environment, particularly in Cambridge now. I think this is partly a result of initiatives to bring researchers together across traditional scientific boundaries, such as Cambridge Neuroscience. **However, I think the biggest US/UK difference now is the prevalent feeling that science is valued much more in the US than it is over here. Despite the best efforts of campaigns like Science is Vital, successive UK governments have failed to invest in science to the same degree as other nations, including the US.** Particularly in the current financial climate, when significant cuts to science funding have been threatened, this means that morale is low, uncertainty is high, and significant numbers of scientists are deciding to move abroad. I don't know that I'm ready to join them yet, but if the situation gets much worse, it would have to be something I'd consider.

Wednesday, October 19, 2011

http://addiction-dirkh.blogspot.com/2011/10/interview-with-neuroscientist-jon.html

Falling Down and Getting Up: Nic Sheff's New Addiction Book

Sheff jumps back on the carousel, lives to tell about it.

What would it be like to have written a drug memoir *and* an autobiography before you turned 30? Would it seem like the end or the beginning? Are there any worlds left to conquer?

The last decade has brought us fleshed-out young examples by Augusten Burroughs, age 37 (*Dry*); Joshua Lyons, 35 (*Pill Head*); and Benoit Denizet-Lewis, 33 (*America Anonymous*). This more or less fits the pattern established by the doyenne of the genre, Elizabeth Wurtzel, who, at age 35, wrote the addiction memoir *More, Now, Again*. And now along comes Nic Sheff to put them all to shame, making geezers out of every one of them. Sheff wrote *Tweak* at 24, telling the world about addiction and how he'd conquered it. Well, as it turns out, not really. But for twenty-somethings, a week is like a year, so two years later, in actual time, comes *We All Fall Down*, in which we learn—if we didn't learn it the first time—that the author is still learning about addiction, doesn't have it figured, and isn't really qualified to give out lessons to anybody just yet. Or perhaps I should wait for *We All Stood Up Again* two years from now before drawing any conclusions.

I know I am being a bit unfair to this well-intentioned young author. I blame it on the flood of weighty pronouncements found in the addiction memoirs that have flooded the market lately. God bless 'em all, but Amazon, by listing Sheff's book as "Young Adult," probably gets it about right. You can't go into these projects expecting great literature. Sheff's text, perhaps in a deliberate appeal to younger readers, is peppered with whatevers, and clauses that begin with "like." His favorite adjective, without question, is "super." Too many one-sentence paragraphs give the book an irritatingly staccato effect at times.

But let's get beyond that. There are good things here, and Sheff is certainly qualified to tell an addiction story: "We stayed locked in our apartment. I went into convulsions shooting cocaine. My arm swelled up with an abscess the size of a baseball. My body stopped producing stool, so I had to reach up inside with a gloved hand and...." And so forth.

There is a standard tension in addiction memoirs by young writers. The dictates of group therapy and 12-step treatment programs clash mightily with their innately sensitive bullshit detectors. **It is hard—understandably—to buy into some of the more narrow-minded and coercive treatment programs they've been tossed into along the way.** I was chilled to hear Sheff quoting substance abuse counselors threatening to commit him to lockdown psych wards, or blackmailing him into signing contracts about who he could or could not be friends with in the compound. **For a free-spirited, open-minded young artist, the distinction between rehab and a Chinese re-education camp is pretty much lost entirely when personal freedoms are arbitrarily limited by lightly qualified drug counselors.** One of the more compelling themes of the book is that rehab, as practiced in many treatment centers across the country, is something of a cuckoo's nest joke. It is a mutual con, where everybody fools everybody in order to turn a profit, on the one hand, and discharge legal or parental obligations, on the other. **"Infallible institutions," as Sheff derides them,**

"that know, absolutely, the difference between right and wrong."

So Sheff plays along, he shucks, he jives, he lies, and it's hard not to sympathize with him as he summarizes one counselor's admonitions: "We don't allow any non-twelve-step-related reading material, and you won't be able to play that guitar you brought with you—so we'll go ahead and keep that locked in the office." Much like prisoners who leave prison chomping at the bit to commit new and more lucrative crimes, these kids are coming out of misguided drug rehab centers with nothing but an urgent desire to wipe away the bad memories of mandatory treatment by getting wasted as soon as possible.

And yet, and yet… **"Once I had some knowledge about alcoholism and addiction, it was impossible to go back to using all carefree and fun," Sheff writes.** "The meetings and the things people told me had pierced the armor of my fantasy world. Somewhere inside I knew the truth."

Maybe there won't be a need for a third memoir. The book has a provisionally happy ending. Sheff found the right doctor, got on the right medications after a diagnosis of Bipolar Disorder (comorbidity, the elephant in the rehab room), and, when last seen, is clean and optimistic.

Sheff does have an appealing, Holden Caulfield-type persona, and this *Catcher in the Rye* mentality perhaps excuses the litany of things in this world that are phony, fucked up, and lame to this endlessly hip kid. All carpets are faded, all motel rooms are dingy. Even his airline boarding pass is "stupid." But the style sometimes works for him: **"Thinking, man, even that cat's got enough sense not to jump on a hot grill twice, no matter how good whatever's left cooking on there might look to her."** Or the time when he realizes that, like any old alkie, it was time to "start switching up liquor stores. That goddamn woman makes me feel as guilty as hell. And, I mean, who is she to judge? Christ." And he's got some nice truisms to deliver: "The most fucked-up detoxes I've ever seen are the people coming off alcohol. It's worse than heroin, worse than benzos, worse than anything. Alcohol can pickle your brain—leaving you helpless, like a child—infantilized—shitting in your pants—ranting madness—disoriented—angry—terrified… You don't go out like Nic Cage in *Leaving Las Vegas*, with a gorgeous woman riding you till your heart stops."

Sunday, May 8, 2011

http://addiction-dirkh.blogspot.com/2011/05/falling-down-and-getting-up-nic-sheffs.html

Interview with Michael Farrell of Australia's National Drug and Alcohol Research Centre

On prisons, pot, and the DSM-V.

Professor Michael Farrell is the director of the National Drug and Alcohol Research Centre (NDARC) at the University of New South Wales in Sydney, Australia. Before that, he was Professor of Addiction Psychiatry at the Institute of Psychiatry at Kings College, London. He has been a member of the WHO Expert Committee on Drug and Alcohol Dependence since 1995, and chaired the Scientific Advisory Committee of the European Monitoring Centre on Drugs and Drug Abuse (EMCDDA) in 2008 for three years. The NDARC does a wide variety of research and data collection on drug abuse, including longitudinal studies of heroin dependence, studies on the prevalence of ADHD among addicts, and evaluation studies of inner city youth at risk. Professor Farrell is a recognized expert on drug abuse in Europe, and was kind enough to share some of his thoughts with Addiction Inbox.

1. Does the National Drug and Alcohol Research Centre (NDARC) of Australia have a specific research slant, or area or interest, or do you try to cover the waterfront?

Michael Farrell: The research base of NDARC is very broad. The Australian Federal Government provides a fifth of our funding under the National Drug Strategy and this includes a brief for national monitoring of drug trends among illicit drug users and improving the evidence base around effective treatment and prevention. Our projects cover the majority of illicit drugs as well as alcohol, prescription drugs and more recently tobacco, and we have a strong international presence through our collaborations with the United Nations, the World Health Organisation and the Global Burden of Disease project.

Our current research programs include prevention, treatment evaluation, policy, law enforcement, health economics and epidemiology. NDARC has two "Centres within the Centre"—NCPIC (see below) and the Drug Policy Modelling Program (DPMP). We have teams working with school-aged children, mothers and babies, and injecting drug users. So it would be fair to say that we are covering the waterfront!

2. You have been critical of proposed revisions in the Diagnostic and Statistical Manual of Mental Disorders (DSM), particularly as they relate to alcoholism. What do you think is going wrong, and what's going right, when it comes to DSM-V changes?

Farrell: The change in overall terminology is probably the most controversial with the reintroduction of "addiction" into the terminology. Personally I prefer "dependence" and think the measurement of dependence has continued to improve over the years. It is important that we use terms that we can measure carefully and be confident that we are all talking the same language. Alcohol abuse and alcohol dependence have been combined into a single disorder of graded severity, the criterion reflecting substance-related legal problems has been removed, and a new diagnostic criterion representing craving has been included. Finally, new diagnostic thresholds for alcohol use disorder (AUD) have been proposed. It seems that there is strong support for the first three changes. However, there is little published literature regarding the impact of the revised diagnostic threshold. **Using data from a survey of over 10,000 people in**

the Australian general population, Mewton and colleagues at NDARC (2010) demonstrated that the prevalence of alcohol use disorder defined according to the DSM-5 was 60 per cent higher than the prevalence of the same disorder according to DSM-IV. A disorder which increases so dramatically in prevalence after applying a new definition is surely problematic.

3. Increasingly, the study of addiction has moved away from traditional medicine and psychiatry, becoming a recognized area of study in molecular biology and neuroscience. How do you personally view this shift in emphasis toward hard science?

Farrell: In reality, no professional groups have been jumping at the chance to handle addiction problems. In the early phases of treatment development it was often religious groups and humanitarian social activist groups who pioneered helping responses for marginalised groups. As the size of the problem and response has grown, thankfully it has been possible to get mainstream health and social care professionals more involved. There is still a need for more involvement. **Modern young doctors need addiction treatment skills if they are to be properly equipped to practice in the 21st century.**

Greater involvement of the biological sciences in the study of addiction holds out the possibility that we might get some exciting breakthroughs in understanding of behaviour, prevention, and treatment. Goodness knows we could do with some new breakthroughs or advances in treatment! A focus on biological sciences does not need to be at the expense of the other social and epidemiological approaches, and ideally, with further investment in research around drugs, we might better understand the interactions between genes and environment.

4. NDARC also houses the National Cannabis Prevention and Information Centre (NCPIC).What is the mission there, and do you see marijuana as an addictive drug?

Farrell: NDARC is privileged to have NCPIC funded by the Federal Government as a "Centre within a Centre" and to the best of my knowledge there is nowhere like it anywhere else in the world. The mission of NCPIC is to reduce the use of cannabis in Australia. Cannabis is the most commonly consumed illicit drug in the country, with one in three (33.5%, 5.8 million) Australians aged 14 years and older reporting having used it in their lifetime. Just over one in ten (10.3%, 1.9 million) had used it in the previous twelve months. The burden of disease associated with cannabis is substantial. I have no doubt that cannabis can result in dependence, and that the stronger, more potent forms of cannabis give rise to more physical and mental health problems. Cannabis dependence seems to occur at rates similar to alcohol, but the effects of cannabis dependence can be mild, and may be associated with otherwise high levels of social function. Equally, dependence at the severe end is associated with significant harms, including poor social functioning and reduced participation in the education and the workforce.

5. You have a long-standing interest in the question of substance abuse in the prison system. Why can't prison officials eliminate the drug trade behind bars?

Farrell: The prison authorities cannot eliminate drugs from behind bars because nearly half of all prisoners have a history of serious drug involvement. **It is no more likely that we will have a drug free prison than it is that we will have a drug free society. The serious gaps in response in prisons are often quite shocking.** The near complete absence of methadone or buprenorphine treatment in American prisons is hard to understand, when you see what a great contribution US research and treatment with methadone and buprenorphine has had globally. Now there are over 300,000 people on methadone in China as part of HIV and AIDS prevention. Most countries in Europe have methadone in their prisons, and many emerging countries have developed prison methadone programmes. But in the US there are only a handful of programmes. There is a need for real change in this area as it is an incredible gap that could be readily addressed.

Overall we still have a long way to go in building an evidence-based approach to drug prevention and treatment. We have come a fair distance in the past twenty years, but the road remains long and winding.

Tuesday, February 21, 2012

http://addiction-dirkh.blogspot.com/2012/02/interview-with-michael-farrell-of.html

Book Review: Writers On The Edge

A compendium of tough prose and poetry about addiction.

Here's a book I'm delighted to promote unabashedly. I even wrote a jacket blurb for it. I called it an **"honest, unflinching book about addiction from a tough group of talented writers. These hard-hitters know whereof they speak, and the language in which they speak can be shocking to the uninitiated—naked prose and poetry about potentially fatal cravings the flesh is heir to—drugs, booze, cutting, overeating, depression, suicide. Not everybody makes it through.** *Writers On The Edge* **is about dependency, and the toll it takes, on the guilty and the innocent alike."**

I am happy to stand by that statement, content to note that this collection of prose and poetry on the subject of addiction and dependency by 22 talented writers, with an introduction by Jerry Stahl of "Permanent Midnight" junky fame, includes a number of names familiar to me. That makes it all the easier to recommend this book—I know some of the talent. Take James Brown, a professor of English at Cal State San Bernardino, the book's co-editor, who offers an excerpt from his excellent memoir, *This River*. James is no stranger to the subject, having pulled out of a drug and alcohol-fueled nosedive that would have felled lesser mortals for good. "Even though you'll always be struggling with your addiction, and may wind up back in rehab," Brown writes, "at least for now, if only for this day, you are free of the miracle potions, powders and pills. If only for this day, you are not among the walking dead." Or my friend Anna David, who is an editor at The Fix, an online addiction and recovery magazine to which I contribute, and author of several books, including *Party Girl* and Falling for Me. Anna poignantly recalls "my shock over the power than booze had... it was the greatest discovery of my life." And Ruth Fowler, another Fix contributor and author of *Girl Undressed*, delivers up a brilliantly detached story of her life as an addict on both coasts and just about everywhere else, which begins with the line, "I gravitated to the fucked up writers."

Then there are the contributors I don't know but wish I did, like co-editor Diana Raab, a registered nurse and award-winning poet, as well as co-author of *Writers and Their Notebooks*, who offers a poem to her grandmother: "Your ashen face and blond bob/ disheveled upon white sheets/on the stretcher held by paramedics/lightly grasping each end, and tiptoeing." Or another poet, B. H. Fairchild, author of the marvelous collection, *Early Occult Memory Systems of the Lower Midwest*: "When I would go into bars in those days/the hard round faces would turn/to speak something like loneliness/but deeper, the rain spilling into gutters/or the sound of a car pulling away/in a moment of sleeplessness just before dawn."

And more: Frederick Barthelme, author of *Double Down: Reflections on Gambling and Loss*. Stephen Jay Schwartz, best-selling crime novelist and former director of development for filmmaker Wolfgang Petersen. Writers Rachel Yoder, Victoria Patterson, David Huddle, and Scott Russell Sanders. Etc. This collection is a rich brew of essay, poetry, and memoir. A tough book, a brutal book, a real heartbreaker with grit. Some people get stronger and rise; some don't. It is a thoughtful and creative compendium of addiction stories, and some of them will surprise you. All of them are solidly written, laid out with an unrelenting realism.

Here it is, these authors are saying. This is how it plays out. Unforgettable stuff.

Saturday, February 4, 2012

http://addiction-dirkh.blogspot.com/2012/02/book-review-writers-on-edge_04.html

Mike Doughty Talks About The Book of Drugs

Former Soul Coughing front man on sobriety and life as a solo artist.

Over the phone, Mike Doughty doesn't have much to say about his former band, Soul Coughing. When I mention it, he gives out a low growl as a warning. He said it all in *The Book of Drugs,* and it doesn't sound like he had much fun. Although the avant-garde rock band created music that was spiky and sneaky and immensely popular, topped off by Doughty's monotonic but strangely penetrating vocal delivery on such classics as "Super Bon Bon," "True Dreams of Wichita," and "Circles," Doughty was drug-dependent and miserable. Musician pitted against musician, egos battered and bruised, credit taken and not taken—and Doughty busily running the gamut of addictions from Jack Daniels to heroin, with a ton of marijuana in the bargain.

But that was the 90s. Since then, Doughty has done two things of note—three, if you count teaching himself German. He has crafted an innovative solo career, and he has escaped from a cornucopia of addictions that had almost buried him alive.

It seems almost unfair that a talented singer/songwriter like Doughty should also turn out to be a good writer, but there you have it. *The Book of Drugs* is informative but not confessional, rock-snarky but tempered with a round of amends. It is also whip-smart and bitterly funny:

—"Lars would go out and get drunk every night, then stumble in, sounding for all the world like he was going around moving absolutely everything in the room a foot to the left."

—"Currently, in the studio next door, guitar overdubs were being recorded for a Meatloaf record. Meatloaf was not in attendance."

—"I smoked three packs a day. Ridiculous. It was like a job. I woke up, and began the work of the first pack. It was a repetitive, manly task, like getting up early every day to chop down pine trees."

—"Weed addicts are along among drug users in that they think their shit is cute."

—"The unsingable girl yelled at me, 'You don't get HIGH, you just get FUCKED UP!'"

Told in an episodic, chapter-free style, the book lays the foundations for Doughty's future by page 3. "My dad's dad," he writes, "was the town drunk in Tullos, Louisiana." Doughty's father was an alcoholic as well. From the outside, the process is unfathomable: Doughty relates what is known as the parable of the jaywalker: "Guy's really into jaywalking, his friends are all like, ha ha funny, then he gets hit, they figure he's done, he does it again, this time gets both legs broke, the friends are like, whoa that's weird, and then he does it again and they're bewildered, and he does it again, and they abandon him, and he does it again, and he does it again."

Here's what Doughty had to say last week in our interview:

—*You got sober after embarking on your solo career. Did you hit bottom, in the classic AA sense?*

The thing that really made me think was when I was actually addicted to alcohol, and I started waking up in the morning with the shakes, and I just had this very logical reaction, which was like, oh, I'm addicted, this is horrible, so I'll just start drinking first thing in the morning. **And that's when it was like, holy shit, I'm an alcoholic, there's alcoholism in my family, and it's not just a "drug thing." It was kind of acceptable to be a heroin addict for me, but it was not acceptable for me to be a morning drunk.**

——Was alcohol your drug of choice, or heroin?

Well, I went through about thirty-five different drugs. I was always good at finding drugs. My struggle was to manage it. If I had to call something my drug of choice, it would be heroin, in terms of the thing that killed the most pain effectively. Eventually, when it stopped working, I'd say, okay, well, I'll just do it on the weekends, or detox for a couple of days, and I'll smoke a lot of weed and I'll drink and I'll do some coke or ecstasy, and then I can be back on the heroin on weekends."

——What's your opinion of addiction as a biological disorder——the disease model approach to it?

I don't really know any addicts that don't have trauma in their backgrounds. I think, to activate this thing, there is generally pain that needs to be numbed, or trauma that needs to be gotten away from. One of the things about the disease model is that so many people of the non-alky variety are just so indignant about it. I think we should just give it up. It's maybe not worth the fight over the semantics of it. It's like, addicts are killing themselves, they're unable to stop using drugs, I would think that would be more important than what to *call* it.

——Did you use any anti-craving drugs, or do any medication-assisted recovery?

I was on naltrexone for a while, but I was getting high on everything but opiates at the time, so it was just a way of not using opiates. I was shit-faced drunk, and stoned, so I don't know what eliminating one specific drug——I don't what the ultimate effect of that was, because for me, I would just go out and find something else.

—*Did you do any formal detox or treatment before you went into the rooms, as AA is often called?*

No. I had a couple of prescribing shrinks and they suggested treatment, because I had insurance, but I was like, fuck that, no way. It's funny, they cover detoxes and rehabs but they don't cover talk therapy. **Most of my struggle to get into the path of non-self destruction was because of a shrink who just nailed me as an addict the moment I met her.** Within probably twenty minutes she was like, "you know, there are AA meetings above St. Mark's Place." And I was so angry, like, "what are you talking about?" So a lot of the struggle, of, you know, am I an addict, or do I just have a problem with a single drug, or are the rooms just a cult, it's a religion—somehow she got me to keep showing up. I don't know what kind of hook she put in me, but I was showing up, strung out, falling asleep in the chair, and she kept me coming back week after week. I don't know what kind of Jedi mind trick she used.

—*You're one of the few performers who have been willing to admit that for a minority of people, marijuana is addictive and has its own characteristic set of withdrawal effects.*

Yeah, my basic line is, if you know a thirty-six year-old wake-and-bake guy, that guy is probably a marijuana addict. I don't know the science, I don't know shit about withdrawal, the mentality of addiction, but I know *plenty* of people that were stoned all day. And they kept doing it. But I definitely believe weed should be legal. First of all, it doesn't make any sense if alcohol is legal. Second, it's such a dirty weapon in the drug war. And the drug war is a war on the poor.

—*You're "co-morbid." You're an addict, and you're diagnosed as bipolar.*

I do know that there was a part of it that was relieved tremendously by meds—a very careful construction of a cocktail of meds by a super-smart prescribing shrink. Really being very cautious and gradual about it. But if I'm really messed up about something emotionally, talk therapy has the most immediate effect. Just being in touch with dudes from the rooms, a sponsor, friends, I'm on a gratitude list with a bunch of guys, we email each other every day—that stuff is a lot more effective in the short term.

—As a polydrug addict and an artist who has seen his way through to sobriety, what message what you like to send to people working in the treatment and recovery fields?

You know, advice is not my scene. I lucked into the right kind of treatment. Something I hear over and over again from people is that they end up with the wrong therapist. It's like a relationship, essentially. I think it would be great if therapists were very upfront about saying, "If I'm not the right person, then let's find you the right person."

—"Don't push against your own weight," you sing in "Diane." It got me thinking about how hard it is for addicts to lift themselves by their own bootstraps through sheer willpower.

If you let go, if you just get out of your own damn way, it will be so much easier. David Mamet wrote a book about the theater, and he has this thing about how directors overmanage plays when they direct them. And his metaphor was that when the airplane was being developed, they had this terrible problem with spinouts. All the time, the pilot would lose control of the plane; it would start spinning and spinning, and crash and hit the ground. So they invented the ejector seat, so if you're having a spinout, you just hit the button and zoom out into the air with a parachute. And they discovered that pretty much immediately when the pilot was out of the plane, the airplane straightened out and righted itself. That's how it is, you try to control too much shit, you're more likely to fuck it up.

—So, things are good?

I'm stoked to be sober. I've got eleven years now. Things are really good, even when they're bad, like a bad year financially or whatever, it's like, oh my god, I'm doing really good. As long as I'm loving the work I'm making, and I have an audience, and I can make a living, those are pretty much the only things I really have any control over.

Saturday, January 14, 2012

http://addiction-dirkh.blogspot.com/2012/01/mike-doughty-talks-about-book-of-drugs.html

Interview with Deni Carise, Chief Clinical Officer of Phoenix House

Why addiction treatment works if you let it.

This time around, our interview features clinical psychologist Deni Carise, senior vice president and chief clinical officer at Phoenix House, a leading non-profit drug treatment organization with more than 100 programs in 10 states. Chances are, you may have seen or heard her already: Dr. Carise has been a guest commentator about drugs and addiction for *Nightline, ABC's Good Morning America, Fox News*, and local New York media outlets. She is frequently quoted in *US News and World Report* and other periodicals, blogs at Huffington Post, and has also consulted for the U.N. Office on Drugs and Crime.

Dr. Carise earned her doctorate at Drexel University, and served as a post-doctoral fellow at the Center for Studies of Addiction at the University of Pennsylvania. Currently, she is also adjunct clinical professor in the University of Pennsylvania's Department of Psychiatry. She has been involved with drug abuse treatment and research for more than 25 years, and has worked extensively in developing countries to integrate science-based drug treatments into local programs. She has worked with adults and adolescent populations including dually diagnosed clients, Native

Americans, and with medical populations (including spinal cord-injured, cardiac care and trauma patients).

1. As chief clinical officer for Phoenix House Foundation, what's your job description?

Deni Carise: My main responsibility is to ensure that we provide the highest possible standard of care. This means making sure that treatment methods across our programs are consistent with the latest research, represent a variety of evidence-based practices, and are delivered with fidelity. I also collaborate on the implementation and evaluation of Phoenix House's national and regional strategies to achieve clinical excellence. My home base is New York, but I work directly with all of our programs and regularly travel to our California, New England, Mid-Atlantic, Texas, and Florida regions. I also oversee the activities of our Family Services, Quality Assurance, Research, Workforce Development, and Training initiatives. Finally, I help Phoenix House spread awareness to the public about the need to reduce the stigma of addiction and to increase access to treatment services.

2. As a clinical psychologist, how did you become involved in drug and alcohol treatment and recovery?

Deni Carise: I actually became involved in the Substance Abuse Treatment (SAT) field prior to becoming a clinical psychologist. **When I decided that I wanted to get sober, I got some help from a counselor. This counselor was so helpful to my recovery that I decided to become an SA counselor so that I could assist others on this journey**. I was working as a model at that time, and there were a few aspects of that career that I didn't like: First, it was very clear that I would become less valuable in my career as I got older; secondly, my value was exclusively based on appearance, not knowledge or skills; and finally, my work didn't contribute to the greater good—that is, no one benefitted by my work. I wanted a new career where I would become more valuable as I got older and more experienced, and where my knowledge and skills would be of value. I also wanted to do something I felt was contributing to society. The SAT field seemed to fit all these criteria.

3.What makes it so difficult for people to accept the disease components of serious drug addiction?

Deni Carise: People have difficulty accepting the disease concept of addiction for three reasons. First, people believe addiction is self-induced; you wouldn't have it if you didn't use drugs, right? There is some truth to this, but of all those who try drugs, an estimated 5 to 10% (depending on the drug) will become addicted. There's a reason why the other 90 to 95% don't become addicted.

That brings us to reason #2: People generally don't believe there is a genetic cause. It is now very clear that there is a genetic component to substance use disorders. For example, if a father is an insulin-dependent diabetic, the heritability estimates range from 70 to 90% likelihood that the man's son will also be diabetic. For hypertension, the heritability estimates are from 25 to 50%, depending which study we look at. **For alcohol, the estimates are 55 to 65% likelihood that a young man will be alcohol dependent if his father is. For opiate dependence, it's 35 to 50%.**

The third and probably most important reason is that people think calling addiction a disease absolves the substance abuser of responsibility for his or her actions. Nothing could be further from the truth. **Those in recovery see the disease of alcoholism or addiction as a moral obligation to get well. If you know you have this disease and the only way to keep it under control is not to use alcohol or drugs, then that's what you have to do.**

4. Overall, treatment doesn't seem to be that effective.What's missing?

Deni Carise: I believe treatment *is* effective.We're just expecting the wrong results. Substance abuse has the same characteristics as any chronic medical disorder. **The problem is that we (society, families, even me) want addiction to respond to treatment as though it's an acute medical problem, like a broken leg or appendicitis.** If it were an acute problem, we could send our kids, loved ones, even ourselves to treatment for a set number of days (maybe 7, maybe 28) and leave the hospital or treatment facility with the condition cured—as we would after surgery for an appendicitis! I would love that.

Unfortunately, we've been measuring treatment success the same way we would for a surgical problem, even though substance abuse and dependence are, in fact, chronic problems. Think about this—substance abuse treatment success is often measured by symptoms, drug use, and life problems prior to treatment and again six months after treatment ends. Imagine if we measured success of diabetes treatment the same way. We would measure their blood sugar levels, weight, number of diabetic crises, and other related problems before treatment. Then we'd send them off to a treatment program where we would prescribe medications, maybe give them insulin, teach them about a good diet, discharge them (take away that treatment), and measure their blood sugar levels, weight, etc. six months after we stopped the medication. Do we really think that would work with diabetes? Then why would we think it would work with addiction?

As with all chronic disorders, there are no prolonged, symptom-free periods without continued attention and self-management of the illness. Just as some people with diabetes can manage their illness with behavioral changes such as making healthy decisions when offered cakes or cookies, or starting an exercise program, some people with substance abuse problems can control their symptoms by changing their behaviors. This means not being around others who use, making the right decisions when offered alcohol or drugs, etc. **For those who can't do this alone, there's treatment**

to teach them how to manage their disease and there are medications to assist them. And I'm talking about the diabetic and the substance abuser.

So treatment can work, but, just like any chronic disease, there's no quick fix.

5. You're committed to working with developing countries to bring scientifically valid treatment within reach of poorer populations. How is the effort going?

Deni Carise: I've been really lucky to be able to consult for numerous treatment systems, universities, and countries around the world—including training clinicians from Nigeria, Thailand, Egypt, Greece, Iran, Singapore, Brazil, China, Iraq, India, and other countries. It's fascinating to see how different countries approach local substance abuse problems. **Some countries have historically asserted that substance abuse is not a problem in their communities, so for them to offer treatment of any kind means they need to change their sociopolitical stance. That doesn't happen quickly.** For one country, the diagnosis of AIDS among 7 substance abusers who had shared needles was the impetus to providing treatment.

Much of what I've done internationally involves cultural adaptations of standardized instruments or clinical tools (such as the Addiction Severity Index assessment tool) for use within various cultures. To do this, I typically meet with numerous staff who deliver direct services in the country. We go over each assessment question or worksheet item looking at what would make sense in their culture. Types of things that frequently need adapting are questions about education (not everyone has "high schools"), employment and income, demographic questions such as race categories, and all manner of expressions used to describe drugs and clinical symptoms. Then we pilot the new interview or service with some local clients and get their perspective and make a final version.

Much of this work has been funded by the United Nations Office on Drug Use and Crime, the National Institute on Drug Abuse and Office of National Drug Control Policy.

Tuesday, March 13, 2012

http://addiction-dirkh.blogspot.com/2012/03/interview-
with-deni-carise-chief.html

Interview with Howard Shaffer of the Division on Addiction at Cambridge Health Alliance

Defining addiction, making research more transparent, and dealing with the DSM-V.

Like many incredibly busy people, Dr. Howard J. Shaffer, associate professor of psychology at Harvard Medical School, is generous with his time. This paradox works to the advantage of Addiction Inbox readers, as Dr. Shaffer, the director of the Division on Addiction at the Cambridge Health Alliance, a Harvard Medical School teaching affiliate, has graciously consented to be interviewed. In addition to maintaining a private practice, Dr. Shaffer has been a principal or co-principal investigator on a wide variety of research projects related to addiction, including the Harvard Project on Gambling and Health, and a federal research project focusing on psychiatric co-morbidity among multiple DUI offenders. He is the past editor of the *Journal of Gambling Studies* and the *Psychology of Addictive Behaviors*.

1. Addiction is not like most medical/mental disorders. If you have cancer or schizophrenia, for example, you can't recover by abstaining from certain things.What's your response to those who say that the disease model of addiction is misleading?

We should remember that the concept of disease is difficult to define. This makes deciding whether addiction is a disease most difficult. However, I think most people accept the idea that addiction reflects a kind of dis-ease. Whenever people get into this disease model debate, it's useful to remember that most models of addiction are misleading, and the disease model is no exception. The map is not the territory, the menu is not the meal, and the diagnosis is not the disorder.

Scientific models are simplified representations of complex phenomena. Models of addiction focus our attention to certain features of addiction and blind us to other potentially important aspects of the disorder.1 **For example, the moral model of addiction suggested that bad judgment was the cause and piety was the solution. Some neurobiological models of addiction suggest that molecular activity is the cause and medication is the solution. Both of these views are simplifications.**

Rather than trying to fit addiction into a particular box, I prefer to think of addiction as a complex multidimensional syndrome – with interactive biological, psychological, and social causes. In this way addiction is similar to other medical, mental and behavioral disorders than we previously have considered. My colleagues and I have been developing a syndrome model of addiction 2-4 that suggests people are vulnerable because of biological, psychological and social influences. **When vulnerable people are exposed to a social context that reliably and robustly shifts their subjective state in a desirable direction, they are at the highest risk for developing addiction.** What I like about this kind of model is that it holds the potential to help us determine who is at most risk so that we can predict the development of addiction – just like we can predict who is at risk for cardiovascular and other diseases. This kind of etiological model will help us establish primary and secondary prevention programs that can reduce the onset of addiction.

2.You have a book coming out soon about problem gambling and how it can be managed. Is gambling a legitimate addiction?

Gambling, as well as most other behavior patterns, can become excessive, lead to adverse consequences, and squeeze out many previously important and healthy behavior patterns. 5,6 Some behavior patterns like eating broccoli rarely lead to addiction, but other improbable behaviors like listening to music, or playing video games might.

I don't think about the idea of a "legitimate" addiction anymore, though I used to. Now I think about addiction as a unitary disorder that has a variety of expressions. For example, AIDS is a syndrome with many different expressions. Syndromes like AIDS and addiction are complex because not all of the signs and symptoms associated with the disorder are present all of the time. Gambling addiction is more rare than alcohol dependence. However, the characteristics of different expressions of addiction and the sequelae across sufferers are more similar than different. Further, the treatments – including the medications – that are effective with one expression of addiction often work with another expression. **Scientific evidence suggests that behaviors, such as excessive gambling, and substance use, such as cocaine, have similar effects on the neurocircuitry of reward – how the brain processes information to produce the experience of pleasure.**

For a pattern of behavior, whether a substance is involved or not, to be considered as an addiction, it must reliably and robustly shift subjective experience in a desirable direction, lead to adverse consequences, and be associated with identifiable underlying biological and psychological features, for example, genetic influences and trauma.

3.You host the Transparency Project.What is it and why did you create it?

The Transparency Project is the world's first data repository for addiction-related industry-funded research. Most people don't realize that private industry funds the majority of scientific research. This particular funding stream is important. However, tobacco industry funded research properly encouraged people to worry that private funding can adversely influence research. In fact, I think observers should worry about the potential bias that might accompany any research, including research supported by public funding sources. There is no warranty that can assure unbiased research, except sound methods and careful data analysis reflecting sound scientific principles. Furthermore, critics shouldn't presume that research is biased just because it has a particular kind of funding source. **We are encouraging scientists who have received industry funding to send their data to the Transparency Project so that others can download and use their data.** This should magnify the value of the data by having others analyze it similarly or differently from the original research. This strategy also should help observers both confirm and question findings, thereby leading to important dialogues about the central issues that are so very important to the advance of scientific knowledge.

4.What's going on right now at the Division on Addiction that you are particularly excited about?

During 2012, we are celebrating our 20th anniversary at the Division on Addiction. The syndrome model is emerging as an important conceptual guide to our work going forward; we are very excited to see that others are similarly interested in this perspective. Very soon, for example, the American Psychological Association will be releasing another of our new books, the APA Addiction Syndrome Handbook. **I am also very excited about our DUI research 7-11 as well as our efforts to develop**

new technology that will help lay interviewers—those often staffing DUI treatment programs—to assess complex psychiatric disorders and triage patients into the care they so desperately need. This is our Computer Assessment and Referral System or CARS project. Lots of people around the world are expressing interest in coming to the Division to study and conduct research focusing on addiction. For me, it is very satisfying to see young people come to the field of addiction with a sense of curiosity, wonder and scientific rigor that have not always been present in this area of interest.

5. *How do you feel about the proposed DSM-V changes regarding addiction?*

By now, most people interested in addiction are aware that the American Psychiatric Association has expressed some interest in moving Pathological Gambling from the impulse control disorder category to a new Addiction and Related Disorders category. **This would represent the first time that the term "addiction" appears in the DSM. If this happens, it is a big deal and, in my opinion, represents a step forward.** In many ways it reflects a syndrome model perspective toward addiction. Although pathological gambling has clinical, epidemiological, etiological, physiological, and treatment commonalities with substance use disorders, my colleague Ryan Martin and I have noted that these similarities also exist among the substance use disorders and a variety of other behavioral expressions of addiction (e.g., excessive shopping). A relatively large literature evidences these commonalities. **Consequently, we think that the DSM-V work group should avoid creating a long list of addictions and related disorders/diagnoses organized by the objects of addiction**. Instead, the syndrome model of addiction encourages an addiction diagnosis that is independent of the objects of addiction, other than as a clinical feature. Diagnostic systems need to identify the core features of addiction and then illustrate these with substance-related and behavioral expressions of this diagnostic class. Conceptualizing addiction this way avoids the incorrect view that the object causes the addiction and shifts the diagnostic focus more sharply toward patient needs.

Wednesday, January 11, 2012

http://addiction-dirkh.blogspot.com/2012/01/interview-with-howard-shaffer-director.html

An Interview With Research Psychologist Vaughan Bell

An expert on abnormal brain function talks about drugs, hallucinations, and addiction.

Vaughan Bell gets around. The multifaceted clinical and research psychologist, currently a Senior Research Fellow at the Institute of Psychiatry, King's College, London, was, in fact, recently down in Colombia for a couple of years. He arrived in the country to teach clinical psychiatry at Hospital Universitario San Vicente de Paúl and the Universidad de Antioquia in Medellín, Colombia, where he remains an honorary professor, but also ended up working for Médecins sans Frontières (Doctors Without Borders) as mental health coordinator for Colombia, which meant that he was quite frequently off in the jungle, doing good work under very bad conditions. Bell has written for numerous scientific journals, including *Cognitive Neuropsychiatry*, *Psychiatry Research*, and *Cortex*. He has also written for *Slate, The Guardian, Scientific American*, and is a contributing editor at *Wired*. The *New York Times* ran a fascinating profile of Bell's work on debunking theories about the Internet as a cause of addiction and psychosis. He is well known online for his contributions to the Mind Hacks blog, which covers unusual and intriguing findings in neuroscience and psychology. He is also working on *The Enchanted Window: How*

Hallucinations Reveal the Hidden Workings of the Mind and Brain, a book for Penguin UK.

Q. *You've been looking into abnormal brain states of late: delusions, hallucinations, and dissociative disorders. Do drugs, madness, brain injuries, and religious experiences have anything in common? Is there an underlying cause for seeing or experiencing things that aren't there?*

Vaughan Bell: Apart from involving the brain, often not. Unusual perceptions occur because the normal processes that allow us to generate sensory impressions of the world become distorted. For example, the idea that we see the world as it is, is a bit of a myth, because we experience things that aren't there all the time. The eye allows light to fall on the retina, two flat areas of photoreceptor cells which provide only patchy and poor resolution coverage of the visual field, and yet we have a very rich visual experience. The brain is filling in the rest. **In your blind spots, you receive no visual information and yet we don't have two black spots in our vision because we 'hallucinate' the best guess visual experience.**

These are not usually considered hallucinations because the experience remains stable and predictable but these same processes, with just slight instabilities, can lead to spectacular hallucinatory states – such as Charles Bonnet syndrome –where damage to the retina leads to visions of monkeys, rabbits and little men. **In other words, there are as many causes for hallucinations as there are causes for our perception of reality.** If the same processes are affected through drugs, brain damage, trance states, stress or simply expectation, we can say that a particular experience has a similar basis but we have to think of the interaction to understand them fully. Trying to explain experiences solely by the brain, mind or environment makes little sense.

Q: *You've experimented with "the vine"—ayahuasca, a powerful South American hallucinogenic plant that contains DMT. You obviously lived to tell about it. Did you see any transdimensional machine elves?*

Bell: There were no transdimensional machine elves, although the whole experience was quite striking. I was kindly invited to take part in the ceremony by a chap called Romualdo, a Uitito taita (shaman), who I happened to meet in a conference about indigenous culture and I was very grateful for the opportunity.

I suspect the experience of meeting what McKenna called the "machine elves" is more prominent when pure DMT is smoked which gives a more concentrated acute dose. The traditional process of taking ayahuasca, known as yagé in Colombia, involves drinking a potion made from the vine until you start puking. To get a fair dose you need to repeat this process several times, so the absorption is much slower. I managed three or four drink – puke cycles and the psychedelic effects were prominent although I never lost track of reality. **I was, however, very struck by the appearance of classic Kluver form constants, geometric patterns that are probably caused by the drug affecting the visual neurons that deal with basic perceptual process (e.g. line detection).**

Q. *As a research psychologist, you have been critical of the disease model of addiction for being both too simplistic about mind and behavior, and too all-encompassing to be credible. In an article for Slate, you wrote: "Despite the scientific implausibility of the same disease—addiction—underlying both damaging heroin use and overenthusiasm for World of Warcraft, the concept has run wild in the popular imagination. Our enthusiasm for labeling new forms of addictions seems to have arisen from a perfect storm of pop medicine, pseudo-neuroscience, and misplaced sympathy for the miserable." How should we view addiction, and how should we be dealing with it?*

Bell: I think we should view addiction as an over-applied label that is distracting us from the fact that not everyone's difficulties with unhelpful repetitive behavior can be understood and treated in the same way. Often compulsive behaviors do have shared factors. **Obsessive-compulsive disorder, impulse control** disorders (like pathological gambling or compulsive stealing) and drug addictions are all known to have shared similar behavioral, neurological and genetic features but that does not mean that each disorder is essentially the same.

The idea that playing too many computer games or compulsive use of the Internet is an addiction like any other is really obscuring the fact that different compulsive behaviors also have many different components. It would be like saying that all "mood disorders" are essentially the same—it would neither be scientifically nor clinically helpful and would cause more confusion than insight. This is the situation we have with addiction at the moment.

Q. You lived and worked in South America for some time. How has the drug trade and the drug war changed that part of the world, in your own experience?

Bell: If you don't mind, I'm going to skip this question. The drug trade is interwoven with the conflict in Colombia and myself and my colleagues in Médecins sans Frontières (Doctors Without Borders) work in areas where the fighting is live and ongoing. One of the things that allows us to do our work in areas controlled by armed groups is that we are a neutral organization solely concerned with providing medical care without getting involved in the politics behind the conflict. Of course, like everyone else, I have a view, but in case it affects either our access to the people we're trying to treat or the security of our teams in the field, I'll keep it to myself when I'm mentioned alongside the organization.

Tuesday, July 19, 2011

http://addiction-dirkh.blogspot.com/2011/07/interview-with-research-psychologist.html

Everybody wants to be Keith Richards

Whereas they might be better off as Patti Smith.

There was a time, not really so long ago, when the growing legion of Rolling Stones fans was divided: Did Keith spell his last name as Richards, with an "s," or was it just plain Richard? Many inquiring minds wanted to know, and for some time, the interesting part was that Keith himself seemed unsure of how to end the argument.

As best I can determine, bringing all my powers as an investigative reporter to bear on this weighty matter, Keith lost track of the final "s" at some point during the late sixties, roughly coinciding with his decent into heavy heroin addiction. However, as the eighties began, Keith, newly detoxed, became "Keith Richards" again, the family name to which he has remained faithful ever since.

This incident is not mentioned in Keith Richards' new autobiography, *Life*. And I relate this story not to suggest that Richards literally forgot how to spell his name during the peak of his several drug addictions—though such things are not outside the bounds of possibility for, say, severely addled speed freaks. **I am, however, suggesting that the Jekyll/Hyde nature of living a life simultaneously in the open and in secret, as an active addict, does exact some form of toll on one's internal representation of self.**

Did the years of the famed guitarist's most severe addiction coincide with the years of peak quality output from the Rolling Stones? They did. The same can be said of Charlie Parker, Miles Davis, Hendrix, and on through the roster of illustrious addicts. Do these same addictive years also coincide with a period during which an abnormal number of people around Keith Richards suffered and died? They do. And this doesn't count the number of people who were mistreated, ignored, inconvenienced, and otherwise dealt with abominably in the course of coping with a key band member's destructive behaviors when addicted.

I knew a friend of a friend who almost died partying with Keith. After a night of cocaine—only the best, pharmaceutical stuff, as Keith is at pains to remind us throughout the course of the book—they took my guy to the hospital in an ambulance, after he suffered some sort of coronary meltdown. This incident is not mentioned in *Life*. Too many similar nights with similar friends to recount them all.

In the end, however, we must allow a certain amount of space to exist between the artist and the art. **As for Keith, I'm a life-long fan. His book is by turns funny, thoughtful, barbed, and observant.** It is a book about a man with addictions, but it is not a book about addiction. In Keith's opinion, the drug problem is a qualitative matter; a result of Thunderbird, Ripple, and bad acid. Here, in one passage, are all the contradictions writ large:

I did a couple of cleanups with Gram Parsons at this time—both unsuccessful. I've been through more cold turkeys than there are freezers. I took the fucking hell week as a matter of course. I took it as being a part of what I was into. But cold turkey, once is enough, and it should be, quite honestly. At the same time I felt totally invincible. And also I was a bit antsy about people telling me what I could put in my body (p. 284).

In the end, this is how we want Keith Richards to be: smart, arrogant, unruly, piratical. Is he, as so many say, lucky to be alive?

I don't know. I have no idea what that means. Some people get addicted to heavy drugs and die, and some don't. If you're convinced you are one of the lucky ones, then I hope you're right.

* * *

Meanwhile, in New York City, a tough little unknown artist named Patti Smith was busily scissoring photos of Keith Richards out of magazines, ultimately cutting her hair and wearing clothes that made her look, as much as possible, just like her idol.

Patti's Smith's memoir, *Just Kids,* which won a National Book Award in 2010, doesn't dwell at length on drugs, either. But we get the drift of Patti's thinking easily enough. Max's Kansas City, the famed punk venue, "was as darkly glamorous as one could wish for. But running through the primary artery, the thing that ultimately accelerated their world and then took them down, was speed. Amphetamine magnified their paranoia, robbed some of their innate powers, drained their confidence, and ravaged their beauty."

Earlier, staying in a hotel for junkies with Robert Mapplethorpe, Patti strikes up a conversation with an old addict in the next room: "He told me the stories of some of his neighbors, room by room, and what they had sacrificed for alcohol and drugs. Never had I seen so much collective misery and lost hopes, forlorn souls who had fouled their lives. He seemed to preside over them all, sweetly mourning his own failed career, dancing through the halls with his length of pale chiffon."

Monday, January 3, 2011

http://addiction-dirkh.blogspot.com/2011/01/everybody-wants-to-be-keith-richards.html

A River of Rage and Redemption

An interview with writer James Brown.

"Who could blame a reader, after James Frey's discredited *A Million Little Pieces*, for being skeptical of the pyrotechnic literature of addiction?" asks Susan Salter Reynolds in her review of James Brown's *This River* in the March 20 *Los Angeles Times*. Besides, it's a cliché to assert that former addicts always know more about drug addiction than the so-called "experts." But Los Angeles writer James Brown, a professor of English at Cal State San Bernardino, is a special case. Brown has a sharp, restless mind, a hair-raising background, and has read just about everything worth reading on the subject of addiction. **In *This River*, James Brown has come not to bury us in bullshit, but to praise the ineffable mysteries of the human condition.** The author writes of the time when, battered and baffled, he clung to the notion of sheer will, of having total mastery over his own destiny—even as the devastating deconstruction of everyday life that drug addiction produces was proceeding apace all around him.

What saved him from dying of drug-related misadventures, like his brother and his sister and a shocking number of his childhood friends? *This River* is no ordinary tale of redemption, but rather a dogged, unadorned, very human description of one man's attempts to understand his disorder, and to find some way to control it.

I asked Brown if he would submit to a brief Q and A by email to be published at Addiction Inbox, and he graciously agreed.

Q. *Recent surveys suggest that kids who had their first drink at 12 or 13 are far more likely to experience alcohol dependence as adults. Did you have any early formative experiences with alcohol or other drugs that in hindsight seem significant to you?*

James Brown: I've heard about this survey, along with another statistic cited in *Under the Influence: A Guide to the Myths and Realities of Alcoholism* by Milam and Ketcham that children born to an alcoholic mother or father have a four times greater chance of becoming alcoholic themselves than if they'd come from teetotaler parents.

Given both studies, if there's truth to them, and I believe there is, I got off to a great start. I took my first hit of marijuana when I was nine, by twelve I'd begun drinking, and by fourteen I had my first taste of heroin. Alcohol and drugs were a way of life in the neighborhoods I grew up in, poor neighborhoods in poor apartment complexes, where nearly all of the kids were raised by single parents, typically mothers.

All the kids I knew and hung out with drank and used. I lost contact with nearly all of my childhood friends over the years, but one became a heroin addict and bank robber (and a good one, if there is such a thing, with over 40 robberies before he got caught), and is currently in San Quentin; another shot one too many loads of meth and died of a heart attack in his 40's; and a good friend, one of my best friends, is still hanging in there. He always loved his marijuana and now gets it prescribed, but he's quit drinking.

So if I'm any example, and if my childhood friends are any example, I'd have to say, based on personal experience, that I believe there is a strong connection between addiction and getting off to an early start at it.

Q. *Tom McGuane once referred to alcoholism as "the writer's black lung disease." Why do you think so many prominent writers have been addicted to alcohol or other drugs?*

James Brown: The list of alcoholic writers is long: Hemingway, Kerouac, Eugene O'Neil, Dorothy Parker, Fitzgerald, Jean Rhys, Poe, Faulkner, and on and on. The only rationalization I can come up with, at least in regard to my own addiction, is spending long, long hours alone in a room, trapped in my own head, imagination, feelings, memories and thoughts, and when it's time to resurface, to leave that room and return to the world that exists outside the sheltered perimeters of my mind, I'd want a drink to ease myself back into it. Without that drink, and the many that followed it, because not even from the beginning could I or did I want to stop after just one or two, it was stimuli overload. Lights seemed brighter. Noises louder. I was expected by my wife and children to just return to earth and join their lives when a big part of me was still locked up in that room.

But these are rationalizations. As the years passed, and the alcohol and drugs took greater hold of me, using and drinking was no longer about easing back into the world but eluding it altogether, where I didn't have to feel or think.   Did booze or drugs help me creatively? No. That's myth, a lie, this notion of the tragic artist. **Outside of Kerouac's *On The Road*, which he wrote on speed, and Stevenson's *Dr. Jekyll and Mr. Hyde*, which he purportedly completed in 21 days spun on coke, and maybe a few other writers, maybe a dozen other exceptions, generally speaking writing under the influence typically produces work that reflects an insensible, messed-up consciousness.** That's scribbling, not writing. Good writing requires clarity of mind and vision.

Q. *Can you describe your experience with the controversial drug Seroquel?*

James Brown: For me Seroquel has been something of a miracle drug and helpful in maintaining my sobriety. As I'm sure you already know it's categorized as an antipsychotic and classified as a "major tranquilizer," as opposed to the "minor tranquilizers," typically members of the benzodiazepine family. Why Seroquel has become a drug of abuse, I have no idea, because it doesn't get you high, at least not for me, and there's no sense of the euphoria associated with Valium and Xanax. Why there's this big push (all the TV ads) to prescribe it for those suffering from depression, I also have no idea, other than the obvious, which is to make the pharmaceutical companies more money. Seroquel is potent stuff, and was prescribed to me for manic-depression (I prefer this term because it more aptly describes the nature of the illness than the euphemistic "bipolar"), post-traumatic stress syndrome and mild schizophrenia.

It took my nervous system about a week or better to adjust, with side effects of blurred vision and garbled speech, but once the sides passed the drug made a major difference in my ability to sleep without the nightmares that have plagued me for many, many years. Also, it made a big difference with the mania aspect of my mental illness, keeping my system at a relatively even keel, but I can only take it at night. If I use it during the day, I can't function well, I can't think clearly or quickly, and I have to be focused when I teach and write. For depression, I use Wellbutrin, which is effective for me. Again, I don't understand, or agree, with the aggressive marketing of Seroquel. It's nothing to mess around with and should only be taken if absolutely necessary for one's mental stability.

Saturday, March 19, 2011

http://addiction-dirkh.blogspot.com/2011/03/river-of-rage-and-redemption.html

Q & A with Nora Volkow

NIDA director discusses cannabis, addiction vaccines, and gambling.

In 2009, Addiction Inbox was given an opportunity to submit questions to Nora Volkow, the director of the National Institute on Drug Abuse (NIDA). Dr. Volkow was kind enough to provide detailed answers by email. In her responses, she reveals a broad clinical understanding of addiction, and speculates on what this brain disorder might mean for "other diseases of addiction" like gambling.

Q: *Clinical studies, like those by Barbara Mason at Scripps Institute, have documented a marijuana withdrawal syndrome among a minority of users. Are we prepared to say that marijuana is addictive? Why didn't we identify this syndrome years ago?*

Nora Volkow: Absolutely, there is no doubt that some users can become addicted to marijuana. In fact, well over half of the close to 7 million Americans classified with dependence or abuse of an illicit drug are dependent on or abuse marijuana. It is important to clarify that while withdrawal is one of the criteria used to diagnose an addiction (which also includes compulsive use in spite of known adverse consequences), it is possible for an individual to suffer withdrawal symptoms without he or she being addicted to an abused substance.

Now, to answer your specific question, the reason for the relatively late realization that people who abuse marijuana can develop a cannabis withdrawal syndrome (CWS) if they try to quit is probably the result of at least two factors. First is the fact (which you hint at already) that a clinically relevant cannabis withdrawal syndrome may only be expected in a subgroup of cannabis-dependent patients. This may be partially explained by marijuana's uptake into and slow release from fat cells, which can occur over days or weeks after last use. Thus, cessation of marijuana use may not be so abrupt, and could thereby diminish signs of withdrawal. The second factor relates to the small to negligible associations between recalled and prospectively assessed withdrawal symptoms, which may have precluded many previous, recall-based studies from detecting or properly characterizing CWS. It is also worth pointing out that other addictions (e.g., cocaine) were also not initially thought of as capable of triggering withdrawal symptoms."

Q: *Are there any anti-craving medications you are particularly excited about at this time?*

Volkow: In the context of nicotine addiction, we have a host of nicotine replacement options as well as medications that work through different mechanisms—all of which reduce craving and the risk of relapse during a cessation attempt, particularly when combined with some form of behavioral therapy. However, sustained abstinence from nicotine has been difficult to achieve, even with the current therapeutics that are available. So, at this point, I am very excited about a novel approach to the treatment of addiction—an approach that relies on vaccine development. Currently there are anti-nicotine vaccines in clinical testing, which are designed to capture the nicotine molecules while still in the bloodstream, thus blocking their entry in to the brain and inhibiting their behavioral effects. And while these vaccines were not intended specifically to reduce cravings, they appear to be effective in helping subjects who develop a high antibody response sustain abstinence over long periods of time. Even those people with a less robust antibody response to the vaccine, decreased their tobacco use. So this approach appears very promising.

Similarly, in the context of opiate addiction, we are very excited about the cumulative positive results of the clinical experience so far with buprenorphine, a long-acting partial agonist that acts on the same receptors as heroin and morphine, relieving drug cravings without producing the same intense "high" or dangerous side effects.

Q: *You have suggested in the past that certain forms of overeating are addictions. There is good evidence for this. What about non-substance addictions, like gambling?*

Volkow: The brain is composed of a finite number of circuits, for, for example, rewarding desirable experiences, remembering and learning about salient features and stimuli in the environment, developing emotional connections to other members of the social group, becoming aware of changes in interoceptive (internal) physiological states, etc. These and a few others are the circuits that the "world" acts upon. So it is almost by necessity that we'll find significant overlaps in the circuits that mediate various forms of compulsive behaviors. We have yet to work out the details and the all important differences, but it stands to reason that there will be many manifestations of what we can call diseases of addiction. Thus, addiction to sex, gambling, alcohol, illicit drugs, shopping, video games, etc. all result from some degree of dysfunction in the ability of the brain to properly process what is salient, accurately predict and value reward, and inhibit emotional reactivity or deleterious behavior.

As we learn more about the significant overlaps at the genetic, neural, circuit, and systems levels we may be able to reap the benefits from complementary research into these various chemical and behavioral addictions.

Wednesday, December 16, 2009

http://addiction-dirkh.blogspot.com/2009/12/q-with-nora-volkow.html

Dirk Hanson is a freelance science writer and blogger covering neuroscience, drugs, and addiction. He is the author of *The Chemical Carousel: What Science Tells Us About Beating Addiction*, and editor of Addiction Inbox. He has written for *Scientific American, The Dana Foundation, The Fix, Salon, Huffington Post, AlterNet, California, Omni,* and other magazines and blogs. He received the 2012 Excellence in Media Award from the College on Problems of Drug Dependence and the National Institute on Drug Abuse for "increasing pubic understanding of scientific issues concerning drug use disorders."

www.ingramcontent.com/pod-product-compliance
Lightning Source LLC
Chambersburg PA
CBHW070627290526
45790CB00001B/27